# Disaster and Emergency Pharmacy

This important book introduces pharmacists and pharmacy students to the basics of disaster and emergency management, illustrating not only the different roles that pharmacists can play within any disaster or emergency, but the practical steps they can take to prepare for these events.

Starting with the UN-recognised Sendai Framework for disaster risk reduction, the book introduces the key concepts and models that pharmacists should understand, before detailing the place of pharmacists within each stage of an emergency or disaster. It also includes interviews with experts in disaster management, shedding light not only on the place of pharmacy within disaster and emergency management, but also the challenges and barriers involved in fulfilling their role.

Concluding with practical advice and guidance, as well as how the lessons of disaster and emergency management can inform the everyday role of pharmacists within wider community healthcare, this will be essential reading for both professionals and students in the field.

**Dr. Kaitlyn E. Watson** is an internationally recognised disaster pharmacist researcher and the Founder and CEO of Disaster Pharmacy Solutions, where she provides innovative training and preparedness activities for the pharmacy workforce. Dr. Watson says, "Disasters and emergencies are inevitable and without proper preparedness, our response will be misguided".

# Disaster and Emergency Pharmacy

A Guide to Preparation and Management

**Kaitlyn E. Watson**

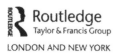

Routledge
Taylor & Francis Group

LONDON AND NEW YORK

First published 2023
by Routledge
4 Park Square, Milton Park, Abingdon, Oxon OX14 4RN

and by Routledge
605 Third Avenue, New York, NY 10158

*Routledge is an imprint of the Taylor & Francis Group, an informa
business*

*British Library Cataloguing-in-Publication Data*
A catalogue record for this book is available from the British Library

ISBN: 978-1-032-41488-1 (hbk)
ISBN: 978-1-032-21532-7 (pbk)
ISBN: 978-1-003-35831-2 (ebk)

DOI: 10.4324/b23292

Typeset in Times New Roman
by MPS Limited, Dehradun

For my daughter, Maddison. May you grow up in a world where you are never told you can't achieve what you set your mind to.

# Contents

# Figures

# Tables

# Preface

*What does it mean to be a disaster pharmacist?* In this book, we will explore this question in detail and learn that it is not a subspeciality reserved for those in a specific position, but that it is an attitude and mindset that we as pharmacists are required to have to continue our operations as a frontline responder during a disaster or emergency. This is not to discredit or takeaway from the amazing work that these pharmacists do that work in these special fields as they provide a great asset to deploying medical teams. But it is to recognise that the premise of responding to an emergency that is impacting your community as a pharmacist is not reserved only for them. Every pharmacist within their community is essential and needs to be capable and willing to step into their role as a first responder.

*But what does it mean to be a first responder?* Movies and television shows have us associating this term 'first responder' with firefighters, police officers, and paramedics. It brings to mind the dramatic scene where there is some accident, and the area is flooded with search and rescue personnel. Absolutely, these responders are essential to any crisis, and we couldn't manage emergencies without them. But the question I ask is, are these three groups of professionals the only first responders? Don't mistake my purpose, I am not discrediting the fundamental and risky work that these individuals do, and I hope if I am ever caught in an emergency that they will be there to help me. But my purpose in bringing this up is to broaden our narrow view of what it means to be a first responder. What about a patient that received a vaccination at a pharmacy and has an anaphylactic reaction, who would be considered a first responder? Only the paramedic that is called or also the pharmacist that administers an epinephrine injection and provides necessary first aid until the ambulance arrives? The definition of a first responder is broadly someone who is among the first to arrive and manage an emergency. To me, this would include the pharmacist as they responded to the emergency unfolding before them. What about the person who calls the pharmacy and expresses suicidal intentions? Would the pharmacist who answers that call and helps the person connect with additional support and care, not also be considered a first responder? I believe this is true for many other healthcare professions, as the same logic can be applied (e.g., family doctors/general practitioners working in the community, social workers, emergency room workers, etc.) and we need to re-evaluate how we view emergencies, emergency response, and disaster management and also who we consider to be first responders.

In the same vein, so often we think of disasters as massive global events, like the 2019 COVID-19 pandemic. However, we again need to broaden our thinking as to what constitutes a disaster or emergency. The definition that I use in terms of health and disasters is – any emergency in our community that overwhelms the healthcare resources available is a disaster and it requires us as pharmacists to respond. For example, an extended power outage that impacts a pharmacy could be an emergency, especially if the pharmacy has no backup generator or emergency plan to enact and they have a large fridge stored with temperature-controlled vaccines.

So, this book is intended for anyone working in the pharmacy workforce, those who work with pharmacists and pharmacy personnel, and pharmacy students learning about the profession. There is a specific focus on pharmacists but the concepts discussed can be adapted to all pharmacy personnel. My focus beginning with pharmacists was strategically considered, as by getting pharmacists through the door, they pry it open for the rest of the pharmacy team. This book covers the foundational understanding all pharmacists and pharmacy personnel should know to participate in emergency management and it is broken up into four parts.

Part I introduces disaster and emergency management, and we will review together the common terminology and definitions. We will also discuss health consequences to be mindful of for certain emergencies, conceptualise the international frameworks that are relevant, and evaluate previously applied disaster pharmacy models.

Part II discusses pharmacists' place in disaster and emergency management, including a look at the history and evolution of pharmacists' roles in disasters. We will also break down pharmacists' roles based on the four phases of the emergency management cycle.

Part III provides evidence from the field through stories and interviews with key stakeholders. This section contains a wealth of knowledge and experiences from pharmacists that have worked extensively in emergencies and we will also hear from first responders about their experience working with pharmacists in the field.

Part IV is a practical guide for pharmacists' and pharmacy personnel working in disasters and emergencies. We review some ethico-legal considerations, how to prepare for emergencies personally and professionally, and I provide some guidance on how to teach disaster management. This section concludes with a discussion on how disasters and emergencies can change us and our professional role identity.

**Dr. Kaitlyn E. Watson**

# Acknowledgements

Thank you to the Routledge Health and Social Care publishing team for taking a chance on me and this book. To Russel George for helping me navigate the initial book and to Leanne Hinves for seeing us across the finish line. Thank you to Evie Lonsdale and Urvi Sharma for answering my endless emails and assisting with the details.

I would like to extend a huge thank you to the experts and people that have participated in my research and were willing to share their experiences with me. I am honoured to hear and to share the stories of the amazing work you do in disaster and emergency management. A special thank you to Dr. Fredrick M. (Skip) Burkle Jr., Dr. Robert Dunne, Amanda Sanburg, and Captain Tim Davis for their willingness to talk to me about their experiences and perspectives of pharmacists in disasters and for consenting to be named in this book along with their interview. I hope your stories and experiences will help influence and change the industry.

A sincere thank you to my loving husband, Chris. For living through and supporting me while I did my Ph.D., for pushing me to keep working or to rest when I needed it, for the endless cups of teas while I worked, for being patient as I continued to say, "just one more minute", and for willingly uprooting our life to move across the pond. You are my biggest champion, and I would not have completed this book without your unwavering love and support. And to our amazing daughter Maddison, who is currently asleep on my chest as I write this, thank you for sharing your precious moments with us.

Thank you to my family and friends for indulging me as I talked about my research for hours on end. To my parents for ensuring I had a solid education in which to build from; especially my mum for being an excellent role model and for never letting me think there was a ceiling above me and my ambitions. The path may not be an easy one, but it is one worth living. To my siblings, thank you for letting me share stories of our childhood and my perspective of being the middle child.

A thank you to my colleague and friend, Dr. Elizabeth (Libby) McCourt. It is a pleasure to work alongside you in pursuing this research field. Thank you for our many collaborations over the years and for partnering with me in Disaster Pharmacy Solutions®. Your work on pharmacists' willingness and preparedness in emergency management is inspiring. Thank you to our Disaster Pharmacy Solutions®' clients for taking the time and resources to further disaster preparedness and emergency management for your teams.

To my Ph.D. supervisors (Drs. Lisa Nissen, Vivienne Tippett, and Judith Singleton), thank you for helping me pursue this topic as my Ph.D., for teaching me the foundational basics of research, and for pushing me to dig deeper into the topic of pharmacists in disasters. I have learnt a lot from you about academia and research.

To my current boss, Dr. Ross Tsuyuki. Thank you for supporting me to continue my disaster research alongside our existing pharmacy practice research projects. I appreciate the support in being able to pursue and work on multiple research studies with our team, especially with the coinciding global COVID-19 pandemic that hit just after I started at the University of Alberta. Thank you to my students and colleagues that have worked on these COVID studies, together we have made great strides in understanding the impact of this crisis on our pharmacy profession.

Lastly, thank you to a mentor and friend, Dr. Theresa Schindel. For reading my book proposal and early drafts, for our many conversations about qualitative research and theories, for collaborating on our COVID research, and for our insightful discussions to develop our various working theories.

# Abbreviations

| | |
|---|---|
| BCP | Business Continuity Plans |
| BGLs | Blood Glucose Levels |
| CBRN | Chemical, Biological, Radiological, and Nuclear |
| CPAP | Continuous Positive Airway Pressure |
| CPR | Cardiopulmonary Resuscitation |
| DMATs | Disaster Medical Assistance Teams |
| ED | Emergency Departments |
| EDL | Essential Drug List |
| FEMA | Federal Emergency Management Agency |
| FIP | International Pharmacy Federation |
| HbA1c | Glycated Haemoglobin |
| ICRC | International Committee of the Red Cross |
| ICU | Intensive Care Units |
| IGEM | Inspector-General for Emergency Management |
| NGOs | Non-governmental Organisations |
| NPS | National Pharmaceutical Stockpiles |
| NSW | New South Wales |
| PERT | Pharmacy Emergency Response Team |
| PTSD | Post-traumatic Stress Disorder |
| SARS | Severe Acute Respiratory Syndrome |
| TTX | Table Top Exercises |
| UN | United Nations |
| UNDRR | UN Office for Disaster Risk Reduction |
| US | United States |
| WADEM | World Association for Disaster and Emergency Medicine |
| WHO | World Health Organization |

# 1 Why I'm a Disaster Pharmacy Researcher? My Autoethnography Narrative

## Introduction

I believe there are distinct moments in life that shape who you are and where you are heading. This has certainly been the case for me and if you had asked me even when I was aspiring to become a pharmacist that this is where I would end up, I'm not sure I would have believed you. So, this is my story of how I became a disaster pharmacist researcher. I decided to write my story as an autoethnography narrative. Autoethnography *"is an autobiographical genre of writing and research that displays multiple layers of consciousness, connecting the personal to the cultural."*[1(p.739)] By using this methodology and technique I am able to illustrate my position as an advocate for the pharmacy profession and welcome you into my perspective as a disaster pharmacy researcher. This is in recognition that all researchers are embedded in their research, and we should acknowledge this premise and our assumptions and perspectives.

## So, Disasters …?

\*\*\*

*It's been two weeks living in a new city and I'm working the late-night shift at the community pharmacy as a pharmacy assistant while completing my studies. I had been working in pharmacy for several years and decided to go to university to become a pharmacist. The shopping centre is quiet with not many people visiting the pharmacy or the grocery store opposite. Knock-off time comes around at 10 pm and we close and head up to the rooftop parking lot where the staff parking is out in the open. It looked like it might have been raining while I was at work for the last eight or so hours as the ground is wet. But I don't really think much of it. I hop into the car, load up the GPS as I'm still not confident where I'm going, and head back to the university where I am living on campus having recently moved interstate. It's my first year at university and I have a full*

DOI: 10.4324/b23292-1

*course load of science subjects with the plan to switch over to pharmacy school the following year.*

*I proceed down a dark street following the directions of the GPS and watching the taillights of the cars in front of me. We drive down a dip or valley in the road between two higher streets. On one side of this valley there is a small park and on the other a lawn bowls club. Next thing I know my car has stopped and there is water halfway up my car door!*

*I am completely flummoxed watching the cars ahead drive out of the water on the other side, but to my left is another car just slightly ahead of me that is also completely stuck. I am beyond freaking out and do what I imagine any other young womanthat has recently moved out of home does, I called my dad [For context: he is in another state and at least a 12-hour drive away]. "Hello darling, how was work?" Dad answers. "I'm surrounded by water, what do I do?" I practically scream down the phone. [Poor thing, I must have given him an absolute heart attack!] "Slow down and tell me what is happening", dad calmly responds. I begin to explain my situation and he's asking me to find the wind-up torch he gave me when I moved out. So, I'm rummaging around in the glovebox pushing everything onto the floor that is covered in water. I found it finally and dad says I need to get out of the car and I'm going to have to climb out the window, with the additional warning of "Don't try to open the door!".*

*"What do I do with my shoes?" I ask. [For context, pharmacy attire is not exactly practical for this type of situation. The uniform including black pants, work button-up shirt, and black ballet-flat type shoes.] I couldn't stop thinking that if I kept myshoes on, they would wash away but if I go barefoot, what is lurking beneath the water. "Leave your shoes and climb out the window and hold onto the car". I put the phone in my pocket, wind down the window and proceed to climb out, struggling to see through the tears streaming down my face. I wade through water up to my thighs and walk the short distance to the higher part of the road. I sit down right there in the middle of the road and watch the scene in front of me. How could this be happening ...?*

*Dad checks I'm alright and tells me to call roadside assistance to have the car towed. So, I'm sitting on an unknown street at 11 pm at night by myself in an unfamiliar place. The tow truck company takes over three hours to come and in the meantime the water recedes and it's like nothing happened, except the car won't start as the water flooded the engine.*

***

It turns out that I was caught in a flash flood due to the storm earlier that night and the water got dammed up with debris in the park and it broke as I happened to be driving past at that exact moment. Talk about bad timing!

It's interesting when I hear people comment that disasters are so rare that it's a waste of time to think or plan ahead for them. I can't help but marvel at this attitude as firstly, they are not as rare as people like to tell themselves and second, isn't that the point – to prepare for the unexpected? Isn't that why we have home or car insurance, with the hope we don't need to use it but then we are prepared to use it if we need to? Or annually checking the smoke alarm batteries, to ensure that in the event of a house fire that we would be woken to crawl to safety. If we only think of insurance or checking the batteries after the emergency has impacted us, how helpful is it really? Disaster and emergencies occur on different scales. I was not prepared for the flash flood that I got caught in. It was the furthest possible thing from my mind but nevertheless it found me, and I needed to respond. I was not prepared, I had no emergency kit in the car, no phone numbers of local people to call to assist, and I was not aware of the increased and known risk of this particular area during a storm. Locals to the area, talk about it, and know to steer clear of this section of road after a storm. But I was ignorant. Hindsight is beautiful thing! But I didn't do my homework and didn't plan for emergencies.

## So, Why Did I Choose to Study Disaster and Emergency Pharmacy?

\*\*\*

*Several people have asked me how I got into disasters from my pharmacy background as very few people would connect pharmacists with disasters and emergency response. After my small personal experience with what it's like to not be prepared, I began my journey of looking for an organisation to volunteer with, once I was a qualified pharmacist. As a new pharmacy graduate, I was finally in a position in my career where I felt I had some control over my decisions of where to next and I have always carried this sense of wanting to help others. I feel genuinely blessed for the education I have received, and I've always had a desire to do volunteer work as a "hobby" on the side of whatever career I ended up in. Anyway, I started doing my research of different volunteer organisations and I even started fundraising for my trip with the all-time Australian classic fundraising event – Cadbury® Chocolate – selling chocolates to my colleagues and friends. I identified several medical and health organisations that were providing humanitarian aid to impacted regions, but I discovered that none of them wanted pharmacists. There were calls for doctors and nurses, but no one wanted me as a pharmacist. I eventually found three organisations that mentioned pharmacy. The first organisation I found was Médecins Sans Frontières, they do employ pharmacists for six months or longer deployments and their roles are mostly logistics focused. But I didn't meet their requirements at the time. The second, was Pharmaciens Sans Frontières, but I was not a Canadian licensed pharmacist, and their roles were also heavily logistics focussed. The third organisation I can't recall the name of, but it was a pharmacy student elective placement in a hospital. Their role description identified that the student would assist in taking a drug inventory as a student-elective.*

*I could not believe after five years of education, degrees, and training in clinical and patient-centred care that this did not translate to being useful in a disaster. Pharmacists were considered essentially logisticians and there was no organisation I could find that would allow me to work as a clinical pharmacist. This discovery flipped my axis, as I had dreams of volunteering on regular trips to regions in need and providing care as a pharmacist. And while yes, in theory nothing was stopping me from volunteering for a general role with these organisations, I wanted to use my education and skills that I had spent years acquiring.*

*Simultaneously to this discovery, I was having meetings with my previous honours supervisor and her team, as they were trying to convince me to do a Ph.D. I honestly had every intention of finding a way to politely decline but my innate need as a middle child to please had me attending the initial meeting to discuss potential projects. They mentioned a few project ideas, mostly around HIV – human immunodeficiency virus – research which while a worthy topic is not a personal interest of mine and I believe you should always be passionate about what you do or study. While we were engaged in small talk about what I had been up since leaving university I mentioned my frustrations at not being able to find a volunteer organisation and how could people think pharmacists are not valuable or capable in a disaster or emergency. One of the team turned to me and said, "I think you found your Ph.D. topic". I was stunned into silence … not something that happens often, I might add. I always thought my desire to work in disasters and to help people going through extraordinary challenges would have to be a hobby as I would need a job to afford and support the habit. But here was an opportunity to combine all these pieces of my identity and passions and not only help people experiencing an emergency but possibly paving the way for other pharmacists to help in disasters and emergencies around the world.*

*So, here I stand on the precipice of my life mission – equipping pharmacists and the pharmacy workforce to be prepared and confident to face disasters and effectively assist on the frontline to help their communities through emergencies and crises.*

***

My Ph.D. topic to start with was focused on pharmacists in humanitarian crises. I was self-serving and wanted to prove that I could be personally useful in a disaster abroad. But what I found was, not only are pharmacists not seen as essential healthcare professionals in oversea deployments for humanitarian aid but even on home soil, local pharmacists were not being utilised in disasters or emergencies that impacted their communities. Pharmacists were not even mentioned in discussions about disaster health issues. I spoke to several military pharmacists as they seemed to be the few recognised or accepted as 'disaster pharmacists' and I found out that 85% of their role was logistics and focused on getting drugs from A to B. Logistics is an important role especially in emergency response and it is a unique skill and expertise of pharmacists, but it only uses a small portion of a pharmacists' skillset. Typically, these deployments that do have a pharmacist only have a single pharmacist and they are in charge of logistics and supply chain management for drugs, medical supplies, blood, and equipment. A few of the pharmacists I spoke to said *"what they learnt at university in the pharmacy degree was 90% not useful for the job they do as a military pharmacist, as they rarely see patients clinically or provide advice to other healthcare professionals working in the field".*[2] Thus, I shifted my focus away from my self-serving earlier idea of 'Australian pharmacists working in humanitarian crises' and zoomed out the lens to see the bigger gap in knowledge and focused on pharmacists in general working in all types of disasters or emergencies both abroad and on home soil.

I had schooledand prepared myself for the answer to the question "do pharmacists have a place in disasters?" to be no. And while I would have been personally devastated, at least I would have the evidence-based answer that explained why I couldn't satisfy my dreams. However, what I discovered was it wasn't that pharmacists didn't have role or place in emergency management, but that no one had ever put the question forward and asked why pharmacists weren't formally acknowledged or integrated into disaster health teams. On the one-hand this is shocking as how hasn't this been thought through before, but on the other-hand knowing the common personality type of pharmacists and how they quietly work away in the background, I guess it's not all that surprising.

History shows that pharmacists have always been undertaking roles in disasters in an ad-hoc fashion, providing care to their patients and communities as the need arose. So, why has noone posed this question before? I think it is tied up in the personalities of pharmacists. I like to think of pharmacists as the middle child. As a middle child myself, this concept really resonates with me, and I can see similarities from my childhood in my profession. Maybe, that's why I became a pharmacist in the first place, subconsciously wanting to join a family of Middletons?

As Middletons, I often feel like we are caught in the middle and struggle with our identity, we aren't the oldest, or the smartest, or the funniest and we don't neatly fit into any one grouping. And this is true of us as pharmacists as well, we don't neatly fit into any one sector of the healthcare system – we are part of the medical team, we are our patient advocates, we provide public health services, we manage the logistics of drug supplies. Like the middle child, pharmacists crave the recognition and attention for the roles and services that we provide. The challenge is we are often forgotten, underappreciated, and underutilised. Especially when a disaster or emergency strikes. Pharmacists have quietly been going about these roles and providing these services unobtrusively in the background, not making a fuss that no one saw them doing it. For example, we have yet to correct the antiquated and outdated stereotypical public opinion that pharmacists "only stick labels on boxes" or "count pills". As pharmacists and the pharmacy organisations that represent us, we don't contradict this narrative. Although we crave attention as Middletons, another classic trait of ours is our self-esteem issues. As pharmacists, we have an identity crisis as we strive to catch up to the trailblazer older sibling whilst simultaneously trying to carve out our place within the healthcare family. We lack the confidence to advocate for ourselves and often our voice is lost in the story. The Urban Dictionary describes middle child syndrome as someone that feels alone and forgotten between the overachieving older sibling and the attention seeking younger sibling.[3] I can't help but relate personally as a middle child and also as a pharmacist, this is how I believe our profession as a collective feels. Research conducted by Rosenthal and colleagues on pharmacists' personalities and pharmacy culture,[4-7] suggests we need to look beyond the perceived barriers to advancing pharmacy practice and look at the pharmacy culture. They propose there are some key aspects of pharmacy culture that need to be considered based on the profession's personality traits:[5]

- Lack of confidence
- Fear of new responsibilities
- Paralysis in the face of ambiguity
- Need for approval
- Risk aversion

Disaster and emergency health management confronts a number of these traits for pharmacists. For example, in the initial aftermath of a disaster or emergency, reliable information is scarce and the supports we usually rely on as pharmacists are not available. This discomfort and ambiguity is challenging for pharmacists on the frontline, as they are often identified as the first health entity to return to operations after an emergency. And yet, when pharmacists are faced with this type of situation and it is impacting their local community, they step through this discomfort and are known for continuing to provide roles and services as required for their community. This makes me wonder, what is it about disasters and emergency situations that causes us as pharmacists to step up in this way? Is it the lack of other services or healthcare professionals available to defer the responsibility/decision to or is it the overwhelming need of our community that we can't help but as Middletons aim to please? Maybe it's a combination of factors that unlock the self-assured, independent healthcare practitioner within all of us to overcome these internal and cultural barriers.

**Being a Disaster Researcher during the COVID-19 Pandemic**

\*\*\*

*While writing this book, the global COVID-19 pandemic is upon us and being a strong pharmacy advocate and a disaster researcher, I keep getting two specific questions posed to me – (1) Did I know the pandemic was going to happen? and (2) What do I think about the pharmacy's response to the pandemic? Firstly, no I am not clairvoyant nor do I have a crystal ball that told me two months after my husband and I moved countries that we would be experiencing a pandemic first-hand. I, like you, did not see the COVID-19 pandemic coming. However, we all should have been prepared for a pandemic or another emergency to impact our communities. Disasters are not as rare as we like to convince ourselves they are. Just look at how many natural hazard events and unprecedented disasters have occurred around the world while globally we have been battling the pandemic (e.g., the wildfires across the globe in Western Canadian, United States (US), Amazon rainforest, or Australia; volcanic eruptions and typhoons in the Philippines; earthquakes and tsunamis in Turkey or Greece; Flooding in Indonesia, Vietnam, or Cambodia; hurricanes and tornadoes in the US or Haiti; cyclones in India; humanitarian and refugee crisis in Venezuelan, Afghanistan, or Yemen; explosion in Beirut, or the war in Ukraine etc.). This list goes on and on. Yet, our coping mechanism defaults to once the pandemic is over, life will return to normal. What normal? These disasters and emergencies will continue to happen and disproportionately impact us and the world around us.*

*To answer the second question I get asked, I am so amazed and proud of how the global pharmacy workforce has stepped up to support the world, during an ongoing and extremely physically and mentally draining period in history. Additionally, I am so excited that pharmacists are finally being recognised as an essential service and for the roles they have continued to provide since the beginning of the pandemic. They did not have the luxury of closing their doors and regrouping with how they will respond to an unknown infectious disease, but they were required to figure it out as they went, pivoting to address the constantly evolving information available.*

*To put it simply, we would not have survived this pandemic, without our pharmacists. In addition to our heavy reliance on their public health services, we have continued to need pharmacy services for our chronic condition management and medicine supply, among a mirid of other roles they perform in our communities. Pharmacists were also a reliable source of mass public health information, provided an accessible place to obtain COVID testing and vaccinations. Globally, pharmacists have single-handedly provided the majority of the COVID vaccinations. All the previous disasters and emergencies that I have studied in terms of pharmacists and their roles has never seen this level of systematic acceptance and dependence on pharmacists to keep healthcare in communities going. COVID-19 is acting as a catalyst and the beginning of a new pharmacy identity and era for pharmacy practice.*

*There is a small part of me that is praying that all this progress we have made through this pandemic won't be for naught. I am concerned that emergency management may be seen as the new 'flavour of the month' but when the dust settles and COVID-19 becomes further and further in our rear-view mirror that pharmacists will be once again be forgotten and left out of emergency management. I wonder who I will be left standing with to continue fighting this battle and advocating for the pharmacy profession's rightful place on the frontline of emergency management.*

\*\*\*

Pharmacists have once again stepped up to meet the needs of their communities during the COVID-19 pandemic. They have continued to provide the steady, reliable, and accessible evidence-based healthcare to the community. My team and I did a survey of Canadian pharmacists and 740 frontline pharmacists responded about the roles they were providing to their communities and the challenges they were facing.[8] Interestingly, over 70% said that their patients were avoiding aspects of the healthcare system out of fear that they would contract the COVID infection.[8] Over 50% of these frontline pharmacists also reported that community members were seeking them out to get reliable information about the evolving nature of the pandemic, and were required to provide emotional and psychological support to allay the public's fears.[8]

The community expects pharmacy to be there during an emergency and to be their communication hub.[2] Patients flock to where they feel safe and secure and research has shown that they identify this with their pharmacy, they see it as their safe haven during a disaster. Thus, pharmacists need to be prepared to undertake their place within the broader emergency management team and should no longer be considered an afterthought.

Pharmacists and others health professions are calling for better opportunities to participate in preparedness activities and for more inclusion of emergency management during their schooling.[9] Yet, when the disaster or emergency resolves and things settle down, this is forgotten until the next event occurs, and the same issues arise. That's why I formed my business – Disaster Pharmacy Solutions™, as a means of providing education and training opportunities for pharmacists and the pharmacy workforce to confidently step into their role as first responders and leaders during crises. These leadership and emergency management skills are transferrable across the diverse pharmacy practice and are not skills that sit on a shelf to be dusted off when a disaster or emergency strikes. Every pharmacy and pharmacy department should include disasters within their Business Continuity Plans (BCPs) or emergency plans and every member/stakeholder in the pharmacy workforce should know what is expected of them when responding to an emergency.

This book provides the foundations on disaster and emergency management which will help you to recognise your role within the system. I encourage you to use this book to help draft your own professional emergency plan and to begin having discussions with your colleagues and workplace on how you will collectively prevent, prepare, respond, and recover from a disaster or emergency.

## Chapter References

1 Denzin NK, Lincoln YS. *The Sage handbook of qualitative research*. Thousand Oaks: Sage; 2011.

2 Watson KE. The roles of pharmacists in disaster health management in natural and anthropogenic disasters. [Thesis]. QUT ePrints: Queensland University of Technology; 2019 Available from: https://eprints.qut.edu.au/130757/

3 Middle child syndrome [Internet]. Urban dictionary; 2009 [cited 2020 August 28]; Available from: https://www.urbandictionary.com/define.php?term=Middle%20Child%20Syndrome

4 Rosenthal M. *Understanding the context of pharmacy practice change: Gaining insight into the professional culture of pharmacy and pharmacists' personality [Thesis]*. University of Alberta; 2014.

5 Rosenthal M, Austin Z, Tsuyuki RT. Are pharmacists the ultimate barrier to pharmacy practice change? *Can. Pharm. J. (Ott)* 2010; 143(1):37–42.

6 Rosenthal M, Sutton J, Austin Z, Tsuyuki RT. Relationship between personality traits and pharmacist performance in a pharmacy practice research trial. *Can. Pharm. J.* 2015; 148(4):209–216.

7 Rosenthal MM, Breault RR, Austin Z, Tsuyuki RT. Pharmacists' self-perception of their professional role: Insights into community pharmacy culture. *J. Am. Pharm. Assoc.* (2003) 2011; 51(3):363–367.

8 Lee DH, Watson KE, Al Hamarneh YN. Impact of COVID-19 on frontline pharmacists' roles and services in Canada: The INSPIRE Survey. *Can. Pharm. J. (Ott)* 2021; 0(0):17151635211028253.

9 Watson KE, Waddell JJ, McCourt EM. *"Vital in today's time": Evaluation of a disaster table-top exercise for pharmacists and pharmacy staff*. Research in Social and Administrative Pharmacy; 2020.

# Part I

# Introduction to Disaster and Emergency Management

# 2 Definitions and Terminology

## Introduction

Now that we are on the same page about all pharmacists being disaster pharmacists and first responders. Let's review the common terminology and definitions, so we are speaking the same language. To be able to take our rightful place in disaster and emergency management, we need to become familiar with the language that is used. In this chapter, I have outlined the various definitions and terminology used in disasters and emergencies that are specifically related to health and pharmacy and are important for you to know.

It's important that we have this understanding and don't skip this step, otherwise miscommunication can occur. It reminds me of those times with loved ones when discussing the need to clean up after dinner. To some that may mean only putting the plates in the dishwasher, for others it also means washing up in the sink what doesn't fit in the dishwasher, some may consider stacking them to do in the jorning, and for others it may mean also wiping down the counters. Does this resonate for anyone else or just me? Unless we discuss the definition or parameters of the words we use, they are open to interpretation and are influenced by our individual experiences. So, let's start off on equal footing and review some of the key terms used in disaster management and emergency response.

## Hazards

Hazards can turn into disasters when they significantly affect a community and exceeds its ability to withstand the impact, without obtaining outside intervention.[1] However, hazards on their own are not inherently a disaster. For example, a fire that burns in an area that is uninhabited by humans is not automatically a disaster. There may be no negative impact and in many regions, fires are a necessary part of the ecosystem and life cycle.

In terms of disaster and emergency management, we go by the definition described in The Sendai Framework, which was developed by the

DOI: 10.4324/b23292-3

United Nations (UN) at the World Conference on Disaster Reduction in 2015, A hazard is:

> ... . *A process, phenomenon or human activity that may cause loss of life, injury or other health impacts, property damage, social and economic disruption or environmental degradation.*[1] *(p.18)*

This hazard definition is quite broad and allows for the inclusion of many different types of hazards than we may or may not typically think of. Additionally, the UN General Assembly separates hazards into three main categories:[1]

1  Natural hazards linked with natural phenomena (e.g., earthquakes and floods)
2  Anthropogenic hazards are *"induced entirely or predominantly by human activities and choices"*[1] (p.18)
3  Socio-natural hazards, a combination of the first two (e.g., climate change and environmental degradation)

Anthropogenic hazards are what we would colloquially call 'manmade disasters', but it's good to know the correct terminology when it's used in emergency management. Universally through risk reduction strategies we are working on preventing or mitigating the impact of hazards on our communities, businesses, and health. However, when this is not possible then often a hazard impacting our society will become a disaster or emergency.

## Humanitarian Emergency

The Humanitarian Coalition defines a humanitarian emergency as,

> ... *an event or series of events that represents a critical threat to the health, safety, security or wellbeing of a community or other large group of people, usually over a wide area.*[2]

Humanitarian crises are grouped under the three hazard categories described above depending on the specifics – natural, anthropogenic, and socio-natural hazards.

## Disasters

Hazards become disasters when they interact with society. Interestingly, there is no consensus on the specific definition of a disaster, as it is heavily dependent on the resources of the impacted community. For example, a hazard that would overwhelm the resources of a small rural community is unlikely to have the same impact on a larger metropolitan city. Thus, what would be considered only as a hazard in one locality could be consider a significant disaster in another.

The most accepted definition of a disaster to-date, was adopted by the Sendai Framework and the UN General Assembly in 2015 and it states a disaster is:

> *A serious disruption of the functioning of a community or a society at any scale due to hazardous events interacting with conditions of exposure, vulnerability and capacity, leading to one or more of the following: human, material, economic and environmental losses and impacts.*[1] *(p.13)*

## Is It Disasters or Emergencies?

The terms 'disaster' and 'emergency' are often used interchangeable in disaster and emergency management, with many regions preferring the term emergency. The rational for this preference is that there is a fine line between what constitutes an emergency and a disaster, and the argument is raised that we should be prepared for any scale of crisis and not only prepared for the big national or international disasters that so readily come to mind (e.g., the COVID-19 pandemic, Hurricane Katrina, etc.).

The challenge with using the term emergency exclusively in terms of healthcare and pharmacy, is we often associate emergency with our hospital emergency departments. Yet, this misses the point that emergency management involves many different sectors of the healthcare industry and heavily involves primary care (although not formally recognised yet). Additionally, for our purposes of preparing the pharmacy workforce, it may seem like emergency management doesn't involve us unless we are working in the hospital setting, which is 100% untrue.

For this book, we will consciously use the two terms interchangeable, in an effort for us to begin to associate emergencies as involving all aspects of pharmacy practice.

## All-Hazards Approach

So, does this mean I'm telling you that we need to be prepared for and have a different emergency management plan for every possible, conceivable, or unknown hazard? No, I am not. I believe in taking an all-hazard approach to emergency management. It is suggested that taking an all-hazards approach allows for a comprehensive framework that accounts for relationships between different types of hazards.[3]

Alternatively, hazard-specific frameworks or plans can often be simplistic and disregards the interconnected relationships between different hazard types. Using an all-hazards approach allows for the development of a single disaster and emergency management plan and risk reduction strategies to account for any conceivable hazard, unknowns, and their mutual relationships to each other.[3]

This also removes the confusion of which plan to enact, making it simpler to follow and execute in an emergency. This is especially true for the pharmacy profession, as the roles we provide to support our communities through one type of disaster are the same as another. It is all an extension of our everyday roles and services, with adaptions required to meet the specific needs of the presenting crisis.

## PPRR

Emergency management and disaster health management are typically discussed in terms of a cycle consisting of four distinct phases – prevention/mitigation/readiness, preparedness, response, and recovery.[4,5] We will cover this in more detail in Part 2 of this book in relation to pharmacists' place in disaster and emergency management.

The terminology used to describe the first phase (prevention/mitigation/readiness) changes depending on what region you are from. Prevention is not about preventing the disaster but preventing the impact of it. This however can cause confusion and thus, some regions prefer mitigation or readiness. Essentially, we all mean the same thing and it is the step involved in taking proactive steps to reduce the risk or impact of hazards on our community. For the purposes of this book, we will use the terminology and acronym PPRR (prevention, preparedness, response, and recovery).

### Disaster Affected

Often people who have been impacted by a disaster are described as 'victims'. However, this can be a restrictive term and fails to highlight the resilience of human nature. So, the preferred term is disaster-affected. This subtle change in language, can have significant impacts on the recovery of individuals and the community. Think of this in a similar way to how we have shifted other health language we use. It is no longer acceptable to label someone by their disease as we begin to recognise the whole person and practice holistic care. As we have accepted the shift from saying diabetic to a person with diabetes, we shift from a victim to a disaster-affected individual.

This term 'affected' is broad to include persons either directly or indirectly affected by an event – sustaining illness, health consequence, injury, or who were displaced, evacuated, or relocated.[1] Persons indirectly affected by a disaster include those affected by disruptions to basic services, affected by changes to critical infrastructure, or who experience psychological and adverse health outcomes.[1] By using this term, we broaden our minds to all those impacted by the emergency and not only those experiencing acute injuries.

## Disaster Risk

There is an acceptable or tolerable level of risk that we accept in disasters and emergencies and it depends on the resiliency of the community.[6] What we aim for in disaster and emergency management is to reduce disaster risk to an acceptable residual risk level by implementing disaster risk reduction strategies. For example, a common fire risk reduction strategy is to have controlled burning or back burning. The goal of disaster risk reduction is to decrease the existing risk and avoid introducing new risks. But what is 'risk'? Well, the UN Office for Disaster Risk Reduction (UNDRR) explains disaster risk as:

> *The potential loss of life, injury, or destroyed or damaged assets which could occur to a system, society or a community in a specific period of time, determined probabilistically as a function of hazard, exposure, vulnerability and capacity.*[6]

One of the major ways we are globally trying to achieve disaster risk reduction, is by countries signing on and committing to reaching risk reduction goals (e.g., reducing carbon emissions, etc.).

## The Sendai Framework

The Sendai Framework was ratified in 2015 with goals to be achieved by 2030. There were 187 signatory countries to the Sendai Framework who all agreed to report on actionable outcomes.[7] This was not the first of these global risk reduction frameworks, as it built upon the previous Hyogo Framework for Action 2005–2015.[8] However, The Sendai Framework has shifted focus to building resilience via risk management and preparedness.[7] This framework is important to understand as it is what we are all currently working towards, and pharmacists are a key to achieving the actionable outcomes. The Sendai Framework suggests that for disaster risk reduction to be effective, emergency management should be inclusive and multi-sectorial.[7] It lists both community and healthcare professionals as stakeholders.[7] This includes the pharmacy workforce, we are a big component of the community and vital for its resiliency and recovery from emergencies.

Additionally, there are four priorities of the Sendai framework. The Sendai Framework Priority three relates to investing in disaster risk reduction for resilience.[7] To achieve this at the local and national level, there is a commitment to health resilience by, *"promoting and enhancing the training capacities in the field of disaster medicine"*,[7] (p.19) and having inclusive policies that facilitate access to basic healthcare services. They outline in the framework that this commitment to build health resilience includes:

> ... *People with life-threatening and chronic disease, due to their particular needs, should be included in the design of policies and plans to manage their risks before, during and after disasters, including having access to life-saving services.*[7 (p.20)]

These goals and priorities outlined in The Sendai Framework include pharmacists. Pharmacists are a part of the disaster and emergency health response and thus we should be promoting and enhancing our training capacities to meet this actionable outcome. Pharmacists are also in a unique position to help address the commitment to patients with chronic conditions. These patients have specific needs during disasters and are often seen as low acuity when healthcare shifts to emergency management. Part of the emergency management protocols, triages disaster-affected individuals as higher priority and those with chronic conditions or the walking wounded as low priority. Yet, these patients are known to their pharmacists and seen regularly by them, so pharmacists should be concentrating their efforts to helping their patients build individual and community resilience. As well as stepping up to continue to provide life-saving services to these patients following a disaster or emergency.

## Disaster Health Management

In terms of health, a disaster or emergency is suggested to occur when there is a misbalance between the health needs of a community and the health resources available to meet those needs.[9] Disasters are complex and require management from many different industries or sectors. For our purposes, we are focusing on one aspect of emergency management that specifically refers to the health implications of disasters - 'Disaster health management'.

The term disaster health management emerged out of the previous historically used term 'disaster medicine'.[9] This change in terminology was in recognition of the multidisciplinary nature of modern healthcare and that management of health problems is no longer the sole responsibility of a single medical profession in disasters.[9,10] The goal of disaster health management is described by Zhong et al. as:

*... to reduce the impact of disasters on human health and wellbeing by providing urgent health interventions and ongoing healthcare during and after disasters.*[11] (p.1)

## Disaster Pharmacy

One sector that is beginning to be recognised as a significant entity is the pharmacy profession. Pharmacists have typically always been assisting in disasters and emergencies but often were working outside of the disaster health management collective in an *ad-hoc* fashion.

Depending on the type of disaster or emergency event, the needs from the disaster-affected community differs and the roles of pharmacists will vary to meet that need. Our pharmacy disaster and emergency plans need to be comprehensive and take an all-hazard approach, so we are prepared for all contingencies to effectively respond.

## Chapter References

1 United Nations General Assembly. *Report of the open-ended intergovernmental expert working group on indicators and terminology relating to disaster risk reduction.* Geneva, Switzerland: United Nations Office for Disaster Risk Reduction (UNISDR); 2016.

2 What is a humanitarian emergency?: Humanitarian coalition; [cited 2021 Jan 24]; Available from: https://www.humanitariancoalition.ca/what-is-a-humanitarian-emergency

3 Lettieri E, Masella C, Radaelli G. Disaster management: Findings from a systematic review. *Dis. Prevent. Manag.* 2009; 18(2):117–136.

4 Resilient Community Organisations. Emergency management: Prevention, preparedness, response & recovery [Internet]. Australian Government Initative, National Climate Change Adaption Research Facility; 2015 [cited 2018 3rd November]; Available from: http://www.webcitation.org/73diZIqnD

5 Baird M. The "phases" of emergency management, background paper. *Prepared for the Intermodal Freight Transportation Institute (ITFI) University of Memphis.* Nashville: Vanderbilt Center for Transportation Research (VECTOR); 2010.

6 UNDRR. Terminology: Disaster risk. United Nations Office for Disaster Risk Reduction (UNDRR); [cited 2021 Jan 23]; Available from: https://www.undrr.org/terminology/disaster-risk

7 The United Nations Office for Disaster Risk Reduction (UNDRR). *Sendai Framework for Disaster Risk Reduction 2015–2030.* Geneva, Switzerland: United Nations Office for Disaster Risk Reduction (UNISDR); 2015.

8 International Strategy for Disaster Reduction (ISDR), United Nations. Hyogo Framework for Action 2005–2015: Building the Resilience of Nations and Communities to Disasters. In: Extract from the final report of the World Conference on Disaster Reduction (A/CONF. 206/6); 2005.

9  Mayner l, Smith e. Chapter 1: Definitions and terminology. in: Fitzgerald GJ, Tarrant M, Aitken P, Fredriksen M., editors. *Disaster Health Management: A Primer for Students and Practitioners. Abingdon.* Oxon: Routledge, an Imprint of the Taylor & Francis Group; 2017. pp. 3–20.

10  Australian Government. *Commonwealth Attorney-General's Department. Disaster Health Handbook 1.* 1st ed. Canberra, Australia: Australian Emergency Management Institute; 2011.

11  Zhong S, Clark M, Hou XY, Zang Y, FitzGerald G. Progress and challenges of disaster health management in China: A scoping review. *Glob. Health Act.* 2014; 7:24986.

# 3 Health Consequences of Emergencies

## Introduction

I believe as pharmacists and pharmacy personnel that we have an obligation to our patients and community members to help them understand their disaster risk and be prepared for any emergency. Part of this starts with our understanding of the different type of health outcomes or consequences that can happen for different types of hazards we may encounter. Not all of these will be relevant for every context, but a basic knowledge of comprehension is expected of us as healthcare professions. For example, knowing the increased risk of specific hazards in the region you are living or working. Just like my personal emergency of the flash flood that I experienced without being aware of the known increased likelihood of that occurring given the storm that had just passed through.

For a little perspective, between 1995 and 2015 there were 6,457 weather-related emergencies accounting for 90% of all disasters and affected the lives of over four billion people globally.[1] The impact of disasters and emergencies on communities is definitely on the rise. And this increased impact is not only from the increasing potential risk of natural hazards, but also due to the amplified exposure and vulnerability of our communities. Additionally, population growth has led to population-dense cities with new communities emerging in hazardous areas, that were historically avoided by urban planners in previous decades.[2,3]

Health impacts from these events can range from minor injuries to death and unfortunately adversely affects those already identified as most vulnerable to disasters.[4] There can also be indirect public health effects or cascading impacts of these events on people's health. So, let's take a look at some specific hazards and their health impacts.

## Earthquakes

A community's vulnerability to an earthquake can be dependent on the amplitude of the seismic waves, timing of the earthquake, and resilience of the community.[5] It is postulated that more people would be injured

DOI: 10.4324/b23292-4

following an earthquake in the middle of the night than during the day, as people would be caught unaware in their sleep and could be slower to appropriately respond.[5] This type of immediate need is best handled by emergency services (e.g., military, firefighters, and paramedics), who are well trained to locate and rescue survivors.[6] The most common health impacts from earthquakes and landslides are acute traumas, crush injuries, cuts and bruises, debris entrapment, and electrocution.[5]

Interestingly to note is the scale used to measure the amplitude of an earthquake – the Mercalli scale. Also, why does this matter? But, it is important in terms of emergency management as the Mercalli scale takes into account the country's vulnerability and resilience to overcome the impact of the earthquake.[5] So, when looking at an earthquake of the same size that occurred in a developed or developing country, the Mercalli scale would take into account the country's resiliency.

Additionally, earthquakes cause significant destruction to homes and buildings including health infrastructure. With this significant infrastructure loss, the majority of those who are affected by the earthquake, end up being temporarily housed in evacuation centres. Research has found that often disaster-affected and displaced individuals arrive at evacuation centres, without their prescriptions or medications.[7] Adverse health outcomes for those with chronic conditions following an earthquake can be reported for months to years after the event.[8]

The glycaemic control of patients with diabetes was studied before and after a major earthquake in Japan.[9] The authors discovered that psychological stress was an independent contributor to worsening glycaemic control for people with diabetes.[9] It was also noted that interruption to medication use contributed to a decline in glycaemic control along with other factors (diet, exercise, and stress).[9] Another study found that following an earthquake there is a spike in chronic cardiac conditions resulting in acute coronary syndrome or acute myocardial infarction episodes as well as increased rate of hospitalisations for patients with ischaemic heart disease over the subsequent five-year period.[8]

## Volcanic Eruptions and Tsunamis

Earthquakes and volcanic eruptions are natural hazards that have the potential to become a disaster for communities built on, or near the fault lines of tectonic plates.[5] To refresh your geography, volcanic eruptions occur when magma rises from the Earth's core and can involve tremors, ash clouds, gas emissions, lava flowing like rivers, and reactions with water.[5]

The major health concerns of volcanic eruptions are caused by the rapid movement of lava and pyroclastic flow (comprised of very hot ash, lava fragments, and gases) cascading down the side of a volcano towards communities.[5] The main injuries that this typically results in include burns, asphyxiation, severe wounds, respiratory problems, and/or death.[5]

When the ocean floor at a plate boundary rises or falls suddenly, it displaces the water above it and launches the rolling waves towards the shore, becoming a tsunami. These walls of water (flash floods) can cause widespread destruction in communities near the epicentre of the earthquake when they reach shore.[5] Sometimes reaching over 30 metres in height and at speeds of up to 800 km/hour, onto land.[10] The biggest disaster management factor of tsunamis and volcanic eruptions are the mass evacuations of the affected areas with the health risks of tsunamis being similar to those of other flood-type emergencies.

## Floods

Unsurprisingly, climate change has seen an increase in extreme weather-related emergencies, especially the risk of flooding.[1,11] Floods and storms have accounted for over 50% of the weather-related disasters from 1995 to 2015, killing 242,000 people and affecting 2.3 billion people globally.[1] Since 1995, floods have been recorded as the most frequent weather-related disaster,[1,12–14] with numbers increasing from 127 to 171 over the period 2005–2014.[1] One of the reasons that flooding impacts society so much, is because of the ever-present need for easy access to natural resources (such as water) which has seen cities built on coastal lines and near rivers, making them vulnerable to flooding.[3,5,14] These communities built in low-lying areas on coasts and rivers are susceptible to floods, storm surges, and tropical cyclones/hurricanes/typhoons.[5]

Floods can affect individuals' health directly by drowning, hypothermia, infections, injuries, carbon monoxide poisoning, respiratory diseases, water contamination, animal bites, or disease outbreaks.[5,12,14–16] However, such an event can also affect individuals' health indirectly through mental health problems, displacement, malnutrition caused by food insecurity, or by collapse of health services and infrastructure, or loss of health workers.[5,15]

This is challenging as the indirect health effects are harder to quantify, and more difficult to link to the flood event due to their delayed presentations.[11,14,15,17] Long term health effects of these type of emergencies include chronic conditions, disability, relocation of the community, and psychosocial impacts.[18]

## Storms

Storms are known by many different names around the world, including hurricanes, cyclones, typhoons, and storm surges and they can often precipitate a flood. Of particular note, is the disparity of impact storms have on high-income and low-income countries. Storms typically affect higher-income countries more often than lower-income countries, however, lower-income countries lose many more lives as a result of a storm.[1] To explain this further, low-income countries had a mortality rate of 89% due to storms for the period 1995–2014.[1] Yet, only 26% of the storms for that same period occurred in these low-income countries.[1] Vulnerability to a storm event is heavily dependent on locality, level of preparedness, existence of pre-warning systems, and the resilience of the community.

The health impacts of storms are similar to other types of events and include acute injuries, disease outbreaks, and chronic condition exacerbations from lack of access to health services and medications. Continuity of medical care for patients who are evacuated due to a disaster like a cyclone or hurricane is essential to prevent disease exacerbations.[5]

Those who were displaced into evacuation centres in the aftermath of Hurricane Katrina in 2005 in the United States, were treated by deployed medical teams. However, the medical needs of the displaced evacuees were unable to be met adequately by the deployed medical teams' pharmaceutical medication caches and consequently, patients were reliant on local pharmacies for medication supplies.[19] Following Cyclone Yasi in 2011 in Northern Queensland, patients who required lifesaving dialysis were evacuated out of the disaster zone, many leaving without their prescriptions, medications, identification, or patient medical records.[20] Medications form a large component of medical care and in the case of Hurricane Katrina, pharmacists and pharmacies were essential in the disaster response.[19,21–26]

## Droughts and Famine

Droughts are becoming more frequent with the changes in rainfall patterns, warming climate, and drier seasons brought on by climate change.[1] Compared to floods and storms which are the two most frequent type of weather-related emergencies, droughts only account for 5% of the natural hazards that occurred globally between 1995 and 2015.[1] Yet, there is a major discrepancy in the impact droughts have on society. Droughts affected over one billion people during this period of 1995 to 2015 which was 25% more people than the total number of people affected by all natural disasters globally in the same timeperiod.[1]

Famine is usually the result of a drought, however, not every drought will lead to a famine.[5] Although a famine can be the result of a natural disaster, there can be other contributing factors related to economic, political, and food distribution activities suggesting famine is more often an anthropogenic hazard than a completely natural hazard.[5]

The main health impacts of drought and famine are malnutrition and communicable diseases.[5] Also, there tends to be decreased health services available in drought impacted areas.[5] With the financial pressures of drought conditions, patients with chronic conditions may opt to temporarily not treat their conditions leading to potential exacerbation and disease progression.[27] This was evident in the drought affecting 80% of Australia in 2018, with farmers questioning whether or not they could afford to spend $40 on their chronic condition medication in light of all their other mounting expenses.[27]

## Extreme Heat and Fires

There are several weather-related hazards specific to heat that impact us including fires, heatwaves, and extreme temperatures. Depending on the region, some use the term wildfires, bushfires, or forest fires. These heat-related events have been linked to an increased risk of illness and death.[28–36]

With the increase in longer drier summers, fires are becoming a more frequent threat as the smallest spark can start a fire.[1,37] There is also the challenge of the finite resources we have globally to fight fires, previously due to the different fire seasons in the southern and northern hemispheres, we often shared resources (such as equipment and personnel). However, with the longer and drier conditions, the fire seasons are overlapping making this sharing of resources more and more challenging.

The health effects of fires can cause potential exacerbation of chronic and mental illnesses as well as acute respiratory distress, cardiovascular complications, burns, injuries, and/or death.[36] However, compared to some other hazards, the health impacts from fires can last well after the fire threat has past, due to the lingering air pollution.[12] Additionally, people living in areas affected by or prone to fires are usually evacuated in great haste and those with chronic conditions will often leave without their prescriptions or medications.[7]

Interestingly, there is no universally accepted definition of a heatwave. This is for the same reason as there is no universal definition of a disaster as it is dependent on the context. In general, a heatwave is defined as – temperatures which exceed the local average temperature for three days or more.[38] This means that the extent of the impact of a heatwave on morbidity and mortality depends on the definition used for a heatwave.[34] Direct adverse health outcomes of a heatwave include heat stroke, heat exhaustion, heat syncope, heat cramps, and dehydration.[12,31,33,39–44] Indirect adverse health outcomes are due to the exacerbation of pre-existing chronic conditions.[44–47] Extreme heat has led to overcrowding of emergency departments (EDs) on hot days in a study conducted in Brisbane, Australia.[48] Individuals ability to cope and manage heat-related symptoms can be altered by things like acclimatisation, medications, and co-morbidities.[44,47,49–51] The elderly population can also be more vulnerable to heat-related disasters as their thermoregulatory system is impaired due to their reduced capacity to increase cardiac output as a cooling mechanism.[52] They have a general dehydrated state due to a decreased thirst complex and their glomerular filtration rate can be reduced making it difficult to conserve water and sodium.[52]

Heat-related events not only affect human physiology but also the productivity of the community, especially in my home context of the Australian climate.[53] Heat effects typically impact city dwellers more than rural dwellers due to the urbanisation of communities and the development of tall-scale cities creating the urban 'heat island effect'.[3,17] These urban areas tend to be hotter compared with rural areas due to land modifications as a result of human activities.[3,17]

## Pandemics and Disease Outbreaks

It is unsurprising to anyone reading this book after having lived through the COVID-19 pandemic, of the significant widespread impact these pandemic events can have on our health and wellbeing. But let's look at some of the specifics about outbreaks and pandemics to help us understand past and future events. As climate change is changing the pattern of vector-borne diseases with vectors breeding and migrating into new geographical areas.[5] It is often unclear whether the cause of an epidemic event was the result of climatic changes in environmental conditions or the result of a failure in preventive measures by community healthcare services.[54] Depending on the disease outbreak, the health impacts can vary from minor injuries to death, but it is variable depending on the vulnerability of a community and individuals within that community.

In 2018, the World Health Organization (WHO) stated healthcare organisations need to be prepared for Disease 'X'.[55] This emphasises that the next disease which may become an epidemic or pandemic could be anything.[55] There are four phases to the escalation of a disease outbreak:[5]

1    sporadic (isolated cases),
2    endemic (disease contained in a community),
3    epidemic (widespread outbreak in a community), and
4    pandemic (widespread nationally or internationally).

Natural hazards can also precede a disease outbreak, epidemic, or pandemic due to the introduction of new pathogens into the disaster-affected area.[5] Our communities can be more susceptible to a disease outbreak following a disaster or emergency, especially if the vaccination rates are low and the transfer from human to human of the disease is high.[5]

## Anthropogenic Emergencies

Another type of emergency which preys on the vulnerability of individuals and communities are anthropogenic hazards. Anthropogenic hazards have a human element and are often believed to be somewhat preventable, including transport accidents, mass gathering incidents, industrial accidents, and terrorist-related events.[56] The health impacts of these anthropogenic events vary widely from minor first aid related injuries at mass gathering events, to life-threatening exposure to chemical, biological, radiological, and nuclear (CBRN) weapons. Chemical and biological weapons may only be identified through the identification of symptomatic people by healthcare professionals,[56] including those presenting to pharmacies. Rapid identification of the agent and dispersal of antidotes and vaccines is essential in the treatment and prophylaxis of CBRN weapons.[56–58]

With appropriate preparedness measures, reduced impact on the healthcare system can be achieved by providing onsite healthcare services for minor conditions.[56] However, any onsite healthcare service can be quickly overwhelmed if a simple mass gathering event turns into a major terrorist-related incident.[56] Taking an all-hazard approach to preparedness in disaster and emergency plans allows for the design of responses for any actuality and the appropriate triaging and scaling up of the emergency response and the allocation of resources to occur quickly.[56]

## Vulnerable Populations

We have discussed many different types of hazards and the health consequences of them, but what makes people more vulnerable or susceptible to these types of disasters and emergencies?

Disaster research has identified women, children, and those who are mentally ill, socially isolated, have reduced mobility, or have pre-existing chronic conditions are at greater risk of experiencing adverse health outcomes during disasters and emergencies.[12,17,59] Neglecting to account for these special populations and providing access to humanitarian assistance after a disaster or emergency is not only failing to recognise their basic human rights but also further increases the vulnerability of these populations.[60]

Interestingly, this was recognised in the 'World Disaster Report 2018', where older individuals and those with disabilities were labelled as *"those left out of the loop: the people we unintentionally exclude"*.[60] I find this both a confronting statement and an opportunity for pharmacists and the pharmacy profession, as these identified groups of people are our patients.

In 2017, there were one billion people in the world living with some form of disability.[60] The proportion of those with disabilities was highest in countries considered environmentally vulnerable.[60] The people most likely to be in need of humanitarian aid during a disaster or emergency, are perceived to be the least able to access or be aware of the assistance.[60] The special needs of older people and people with disabilities, including medications for their chronic conditions are often not prioritised in disasters.[60] But this is an area that pharmacists and the pharmacy profession can make a big impact.

So, let's look at some of these special populations in more details.

### Older Individuals

In 2017, 8% of the world's population were over the age of 60.[60] By the year 2100, this is expected to increase to 22% of the projected world's population.[60] But let's not jump the gun here, ageing along does not necessarily increase a person's vulnerability.[61] To be considered more vulnerable, older age needs to be combined with some form of physical, social, cognitive, economic, or psychological circumstance that inhibits their ability to respond to a disaster.[61] This is often the case with older people that have reduced mobility, social isolation, discrimination, and their increased likelihood of chronic conditions.[60] However, it is not always the case.

### Individuals with Chronic Conditions

Globally, it is suggested that as many as one in five people have multiple chronic conditions and with the ageing population and obesity trends, this is expected to escalate in the coming years.[62] The interruption to essential services significantly hinders an affected community's ability to recover after a disaster or emergency.[63] This is even more pronounced for people living with chronic conditions that rely on these services.

Individuals with chronic conditions can develop complications during disasters and represent the most prevalent adversely affected group.[5,64] Disaster health research has identified diabetes, cancer, chronic respiratory diseases (chronic obstructive pulmonary disease and asthma), cardiovascular disease, and kidney disease as the five most common chronic conditions that are exacerbated during weather-related disasters and emergencies.[65–69] Some individuals (e.g., those who have had an organ transplant or who are immunocompromised) are also at increased risk of contracting a communicable disease in the aftermath of a disaster or emergency.[65]

As you I'm sure are aware, patients with chronic conditions require a multitude of healthcare professionals and medications to effectively manage their conditions and prevent disease progression. Individuals with chronic conditions rely heavily on essential healthcare services to optimally manage their conditions (e.g., specific medical equipment (e.g., nebulisers, oxygen machines, continuous positive airway pressure (CPAP) machines, dialysis machines, insulin pumps, blood glucose levels (BGLs) monitors, and blood pressure monitors), others require care involving in-home services, and some of their treatments must be given on a strict schedule).[61,65,69] However, during emergencies these services are not always available. Primary and secondary healthcare systems can collapse,[70] and tertiary healthcare systems (e.g., hospitals) become overcrowded and follow emergency protocols focused on acutely injured disaster-affected indivduals.[61]

For example, patients with chronic kidney disease are prescribed numerous medications, and some require dialysis multiple times a week.[71] These patients cannot go without dialysis or their medications for very long. Dialysis requires continuous power, clean water, equipment, and trained personnel.[72] These resources may not be readily available during a disaster or emergency.[20] Additionally, patients with chronic kidney disease must keep to a strict diet of low protein, potassium, sodium, and phosphate and are placed on fluid restrictions.[20,64,73]

Another common chronic condition that is impacted is – diabetes mellitus. Diabetes mellitus can be challenging with patients taking multiple medications and needing to test their BGLs regularly. Research has shown glycaemic control and glycated haemoglobin (HbA1c) levels (the clinical parameters for diabetes control) become elevated following disasters increasing patients' risk of developing complications.[9,64,74] Patients with diabetes mellitus need to consume a modified, controlled amount of carbohydrates and sugars in their diet, and eat regularly to sustain their insulin and sugar balance.[65,75] Appropriate food and lifesaving insulin medication may not be readily available during or following a disaster, and the potential adverse health outcomes can be life-threatening.[65]

In many disaster situations, food drops and evacuation centres do not have tailored packages for those requiring a specific, tailored diet.[65,76] With so many people in a community affected by a disaster or emergency, governments and humanitarian aid organisations attempt to help the larger majority of people and this is achieved by giving generalised assistance (i.e., looking at the community's needs as a whole).[76] The concerning factor with providing standardised care in the wake of an emergency is the rise in chronic conditions occurring globally and the specialised needs of some of these patient groups.

Sadly, post-disaster health trends have seen an uptake in smoking, alcohol consumption, poor diets, and poor sleeping habits due to the high stress, and can be associated with post-traumatic stress disorder (PTSD).[8,77] These habits are risk factors for cardiovascular-related diseases as well as other chronic diseases such as diabetes.[8,77] PTSD has been previouslylinked to an increase in newly diagnosed Type 2 Diabetes Mellitus.[77] This link between PTSD and Type 2 Diabetes Mellitus could be the result of individuals with PTSD being treated with second generation antipsychotics, the side effects which include metabolic syndrome and diabetes.[77] It could also be the result of poor lifestyle habits undertaken following a disaster or emergency which are generally associated with PTSD.[77]

## Continuity of Medication Management

As I mentioned before during disasters and emergencies, the healthcare system changes its focus and priorities, going into a 'state of emergency' management. This includes personnel and resources being redeployed or reallocated to accommodate the influx of disaster-related injuries expected. Disaster studies have reported that emergency services and hospitals are inundated with a surge of patients following a disaster, but few of the presenting individuals actually require acute emergency care.[21–23,78] Most simply lack an alternative to address their non-acute medical concerns.[21–23,78] This causes a significant overcrowding of hospitals and EDs that are already struggling to allocate the limited healthcare resources available to them. A simulated exercise carried out in the United States of a plague epidemic, identified the hospitals involved were beyond capacity within 24 hours, some receiving 10 times their normal volume of patients.[79]

The principal observation from disaster health literature is that patients with chronic conditions affected by disasters struggle to obtain supply of their medications – many of which are lifesaving and even a single dose cannot be missed.[7,65,68,75] In 2014, a systematic review was conducted and the authors discovered medication refills from lost or destroyed medications places a huge burden on the healthcare teams responding to emergencies.[7] The study found evacuees require not only lifesaving and essential medications following a disaster event but also other medical-related items.[7] These include glasses, hearing aids, insulin pens and needles, walkers, canes and wheelchairs, CPAP machines, oxygen machines, nebulisers, nutritional supplements for tube feeding, dentures, and dosage administration aids.[7] Many of these items can be supplied by most community pharmacies.

The interruption to ongoing medication management can be attributed to a number of reasons – no access to a pharmacy, no prescription, contaminated medications, no money to pay for medications, no identification, or people's unwillingness to go to the overcrowded hospitals or venture out into the disaster-affected areas.[68,75,80] Many individuals who are evacuated leave their homes without their medications or they are lost, destroyed by contaminated water, or extreme heat.[25] While for others it can be a matter of financial burden of needing to replace their medications and being unable to afford new supplies. Interestingly, a study conducted in the United States in 2013 found that insurance companies believe it is pharmacists' responsibility to ensure patients have access to continuity of care in the event of a disaster.[67] However, these insurance companies were unwilling to discuss entering into an agreement which gave patients access to their chronic medications earlier to build a personal reserve in the event of a disaster.[67] Perhaps, this is an area for our pharmacy advocacy bodies and organisations to advocate for change.

A patients' loss of identification and medical records during emergencies can also have a significant impact on the continuity of their medication supply.[7,72] Lack of records and identification means medication supply becomes reliant on physician's repeating and confirming the patient's diagnosis or patients' recollection and memory of their medications' names, doses, and strengths.[20,65,68] Disaster research from evacuation centres in New Orleans, United States, in the wake of Hurricane Katrina, reported that 56.7% of patients requiring medical assistance needed prescriptions for chronic conditions medications.[21]

## Chapter References

1 Centre for Research on the Epidemiology of Disasters (CRED). United Nations Office for Disaster Risk Reduction (UNISDR). The Human Cost of Weather-Related Disasters 1995-2015. Brussels, Belgium. Geneva, Switzerland 2015.

2 Mercer J, Dominey-Howes D, Kelman I, Lloyd K. The potential for combining indigenous and western knowledge in reducing vulnerability to environmental hazards in small island developing states. *Environ. Haz.* 2007; 7(4):245–256.

3 Campbell-Lendrum D, Corvalán C. Climate change and developing-country cities: Implications for environmental health and equity. *J. Urban Health* 2007; 84(1):109–117.

4 Ryan B, Franklin R. Chapter 2: Disaster trends and impact. In: FitzGerald GJ, Tarrant M, Aitken P, Fredriksen M, editors. *Disaster health management: A primer for students and practitioners. Abingdon.* Oxon: Routledge, an imprint of the Taylor & Francis Group; 2017. p. 21–36.

5 Chan EYY. *Public health humanitarian responses to natural disasters.* Taylor & Francis; 2017.

6 Zhang L, Liu X, Li Y, Liu Y, Liu Z, Lin J, et al. Emergency medical rescue efforts after a major earthquake: Lessons from the 2008 Wenchuan earthquake. *Lancet (London, England)* 2012; 379(9818):853–861.

7 Ochi SHS, Landeg O, Mayner L, Murray V. Disaster-driven evacuation and medication loss: A systematic literature review. *PLoS Curr. Dis.* 2014; 6:1–20.

8 Huang K, Huang D, He D, Van Loenhout J, Liu W, Huang B, et al. Changes in hospitalization for ischemic heart disease after the 2008 Sichuan earthquake: 10 years of data in a population of 300,000. *Disaster Med. Public Health Prep* 2016; 10(02):203–210.

9 Fujihara K, Saito A, Heianza Y, Gibo H, Suzuki H, Shimano H, et al. Impact of psychological stress caused by the Great East Japan earthquake on glycemic control in patients with diabetes. *Exp. Clin. Endocrinol. Diabetes* 2012; 120(09):560–563.

10 National Geographic. Tsunamis 101 [Internet]. National Geographic Partners, LLC; [cited 2018 27th Oct]; Available from: http://www.webcitation. org/73TKlnSB3

11 Ahern M, Kovats RS, Wilkinson P, Few R, Matthies F. Global health impacts of floods: Epidemiologic evidence. *Epidemiol. Rev.* 2005; 27(1):36–46.

12 Smith KR, Woodward A, Campbell-Lendrum D, Chadee D, Honda Y, Liu Q, et al. *Human health: Impacts, adaptation, and co-benefits. In: Climate change 2014: Impacts, adaptation, and vulnerability. Part A: Global and Sectoral Aspects. Contribution of Working Group II to the Fifth Assessment Report of the Intergovernmental Panel on Climate Change.* [Field CB, Barros VR, Dokken DJ, Mach KJ, Mastrandrea MD, Bilir TE, Chatterjee M, Ebi KL, Estrada YO, Genova RC, Girma B, Kissel ES, Levy AN, MacCracken S, Mastrandrea PR, and White LL, (eds.)]. Cambridge, United Kingdom and New York, NY, USA: Cambridge University Press; 2014. p. 709–754.

13 Guha-Sapir D, Hoyois P. *Estimating populations affected by disasters: A review of methodological issues and research gaps. Centre for Research on the Epidemiology of Disasters (CRED).* Brussels: Institute of Health and Society (IRSS), Université catholique de Louvain; 2015.

14 Du W, FitzGerald GJ, Clark M, Hou XY. Health impacts of floods. *Prehosp. Disaster Med.* 2010; 25(3):265–272.

15 Handmer J, Honda Y, Kundzewicz ZW, Arnell N, Benito G, Hatfield J, et al. Changes in impacts of climate extremes: Human systems and ecosystems. In: *Managing the risks of extreme events and disasters to advance climate change adaptation. A Special Report Of Working Groups I And II Of The Intergovernmental Panel On Climate Change.* Cambridge, UK and New York, NY, USA: Cambridge University Press; 2012. p. 231–290.

16 Frumkin H, Hess J, Luber G, Malilay J, McGeehin M. Climate change: The public health response. *Am. J. Public Health* 2008; 98(3):435–445.

17 McMichael AJ, Woodruff RE, Hales S. Climate change and human health: Present and future risks. *Lancet (London, England)* 2006; 367(9513):859–869.

18 Zhong S, Yang L, Toloo S, Wang Z, Tong S, Sun X, et al. The long-term physical and psychological health impacts of flooding: A systematic mapping. *Sci. Total Environ* 2018; 626:165–194.

19 Jhung MA, Shehab N, Rohr-Allegrini C, Pollock DA, Sanchez R, Guerra F, et al. Chronic disease and disasters. Medication demands of hurricane Katrina evacuees. *Am. J. Prev. Med.* 2007; 33(3):207–210.

20 Rossi M, Young V, Martin J, Douglas B, Campbell K. Nutrition during a natural disaster for people with end-stage kidney disease. *Renal Society of Australasia Journal* 2011; 7(2):69–71.

21 Currier M, King DS, Wofford MR, Daniel BJ. A Katrina experience: Lessons learned. *Am. J. Med.* 2006; 119(11):986–992.

22 Traynor K. Pharmacy, public health intersect in Alabama disaster plans. *Am. J. Health Syst. Pharm.* 2007; 64(19):1998–1999.

23 Hogue MD, Hogue HB, Lander RD, Avent K, Fleenor M. The non traditional role of pharmacists after Hurricane Katrina: Process description and lessons learned. *Public Health Rep.* 2009; 124(2):217–223.

24 Young D. Pharmacists play vital roles in Katrina response more disaster-response participation urged. *Am. J. Health Syst. Pharm.* 2005; 62(21): 2202–2216.

25 Velazquez L, Dallas S, Rose L, Eva KS, Saville R, Wang J, et al. A PHS pharmacist team's response to Hurricane Katrina. *Am. J. Health Syst. Pharm.* 2006; 63(14).

26 Bratberg J. Hurricane Katrina: Pharmacists making a difference: A Rhode Island pharmacist shares his gulf coast experiences as part of a disaster-relief team. *J. Am. Pharm. Assoc.* (2003) 2005; 45(6):654–658.

27 Brooker C. Drought breaker. AJP: The Australian Journal of Pharmacy 2018.

28 Xiao J, Spicer T, Jian L, Yun GY, Shao C, Nairn J, et al. Variation in population vulnerability to heat wave in Western Australia. *Front Public Health* 2017; 5:64.

29 Basu R. High ambient temperature and mortality: A review of epidemiologic studies from 2001 to 2008. *Environ. Health* 2009; 8(1):40.

30 Basu R, Samet JM. Relation between elevated ambient temperature and mortality: A review of the epidemiologic evidence. *Epidemiol. Rev.* 2002; 24(2):190–202.

31 Kovats RS, Hajat S. Heat stress and public health: A critical review. *Annu. Rev. Public Health* 2008; 29(1):41–55.

32 O'Neill MS, Ebi KL. Temperature extremes and health: Impacts of climate variability and change in the United States. *J. Occup. Environ. Med.* 2009; 51(1):13–25.

33 Bi P, Williams S, Loughnan M, Lloyd G, Hansen A, Kjellstrom T, et al. The effects of extreme heat on human mortality and morbidity in Australia: Implications for public health. *Asia Pac. J. Public Health* 2011; 23(2):27S–36S.

34 Xu Z, Fitzgerald G, Guo Y, Jalaludin B, Tong S. Impact of heatwave on mortality under different heatwave definitions: A systematic review and meta-analysis. *Environ. Int.* 2016; 89–90(C):193–203.

35 Johnston FH. Bushfires and human health in a changing environment. *Aust. Fam. Physician* 2009; 38(9):720–724.

36 Liu JC, Pereira G, Uhl SA, Bravo MA, Bell ML. A systematic review of the physical health impacts from non-occupational exposure to wildfire smoke. *Environ. Res.* 2015; 136:120–132.

37 Intergovernmental Panel on Climate Change (IPCC) Climate change: New dimensions in disaster risk, exposure, vulnerability, and resilience. In: Lavell A, Oppenheimer M, Diop C, Hess J, Lempert R, Li J, et al., editors. *Managing the risks of extreme events and disasters to advance climate change adaptation. A Special Report of Working Groups I and II of the Intergovernmental Panel on Climate Change.* Cambridge, UK, and New York, NY, USA: Cambridge University Press; 2012. p. 25–64.

38 Tong S, Wang XY, Barnett AG. Assessment of heat-related health impacts in Brisbane, Australia: Comparison of different heatwave definitions. *PLoS One* 2010; 5(8):e12155.

39 Semenza JC, McCullough JE, Flanders WD, McGeehin MA, Lumpkin JR. excess hospital admissions during the July 1995 heat wave in Chicago. *Am. J. Prev. Med.* 1999; 16(4):269–277.

40 Herbst J, Mason K, Byard RW, Gilbert JD, Charlwood C, Heath KJ, et al. Heat-related deaths in Adelaide, South Australia: Review of the literature and case findings–An Australian perspective. *J. Forensic Leg. Med.* 2014; 22:73–78.

41 Jones TS, Choi K, Thacker SB, Liang AP, Kilbourne EM, Griffin MR, et al. Morbidity and mortality associated with the July 1980 heat wave in St Louis and Kansas City, Mo. *JAMA.* 1982; 247(24):3327–3331.

42  Kilbourne EM. The spectrum of illness during heat waves. *Am. J. Prev. Med.* 1999; 16(4):359.

43  Langlois N, Herbst J, Mason K, Nairn J, Byard RW. Using the excess heat factor (EHF) to predict the risk of heat related deaths. J. *Forensic Leg. Med.* 2013; 20(5):408–411.

44  McGeehin MA, Mirabelli M. The potential impacts of climate variability and change on temperature-related morbidity and mortality in the United States. *Environ. Health Perspect.* 2001; 109(Suppl 2):185–189.

45  Hales S, Edwards S, Kovats RS, A McMichael D, Campbell-Lendrum C, Corvalán K, et al. Impacts on health of climate extremes. In: *Climate change and human health: Risks and response.* Geneva: World Health Organization; 2003. p. 79–102.

46  Kilbourne EM. *Heat waves and hot environments.* New York: Oxford University Press; 1997.

47  Kravchenko J, Abernethy AP, Fawzy M, Lyerly HK. Minimization of heat-wave morbidity and mortality. *Am. J. Prev. Med.* 2013; 44(3):274–282.

48  Toloo GS, Hu W, Fitzgerald G, Aitken P, Tong S. Projecting excess emergency department visits and associated costs in Brisbane, Australia, Under population growth and climate change scenarios. *Sci. Rep.* 2015; 5(1):12860.

49  Nitschke M, Tucker GR, Bi P. Morbidity and mortality during heatwaves in metropolitan Adelaide. *Med. J. Aust.* 2007; 187(11–12):662.

50  Nitschke M, Tucker GR, Hansen AL, Williams S, Zhang Y, Bi P. Impact of two recent extreme heat episodes on morbidity and mortality in Adelaide, South Australia: A case-series analysis. *Environ. Health* 2011; 10(1):42.

51  Stafoggia M, De Maria M, Michelozzi P, Miglio R, Pandolfi P, Picciotto S, et al. Vulnerability to heat-related mortality: A multicity, population-based, case-crossover analysis. *Epidemiology* 2006; 17(3):315–323.

52  Horton G, Hanna L, Kelly B. Drought, drying and climate change: Emerging health issues for ageing Australians in rural areas. *Australas. J. Ageing* 2010; 29(1):2–7.

53  Sauerborn R, Kjellstrom T, Nilsson M. Invited editorial: Health as a crucial driver for climate policy. *Glob Health Action* 2009; 2.

54  McMichael AJ. *Climate change and human health: Risks and responses.* World Health Organization; 2003.

55  World Health Organization. *2018 Annual review of diseases prioritized under the research and development blueprint.* Geneva, Switzerland; 2018.

56  Oh C, Mazar S, Logan P. Chapter 21: Manmade disasters. In: FitzGerald GJ, Tarrant M, Aitken P, Fredriksen M, editors. *Disaster health management: A primer for students and practitioners.* Abingdon, Oxon: Routledge, an imprint of the Taylor & Francis Group; 2017. p. 267–281.

57  Anderson PD. Emergency management of chemical weapons injuries. *J. Pharm. Pract* 2012; 25(1):61–68.

58  Burda AM, Sigg T. Pharmacy preparedness for incidents involving weapons of mass destruction. *J. Pharm. Pract.* 2000; 13(2):141–155.

59  Mokdad AH, Mensah GA, Posner SF, Reed E, Simoes EJ, Engelgau M, et al. When chronic conditions become acute: Prevention and control of chronic diseases and adverse health outcomes during natural disasters. *Prev. Chronic Dis.* 2005; 2(Suppl 1):A04.

60 The International Federation of Red Cross and Red Crescent Societies. World Disaster Report 2018. Leaving no-one behind: The international humanitarian sector must do more to respond to the needs of the world's most vulnerable people. Geneva, Switzerland; 2018.

61 Fernandez LS, Byard D, Lin C-C, Benson S, Barbera JA. Frail elderly as disaster victims: Emergency management strategies. *Prehosp. Disaster Med.* 2002; 17(02):67–74.

62 Mossialos E, Courtin E, Naci H, Benrimoj S, Bouvy M, Farris K, et al. From "retailers" to health care providers: Transforming the role of community pharmacists in chronic disease management. *Health Policy* 2015; 119(5): 628–639.

63 Australian Business Roundtable for Disaster Resilience and Safer Communities. Building our nation's resilience to natural disasters. *Deloitte Access Economics* 2013. Deloitte Access Economics Barton, ACT.

64 Miller AC, Arquilla B. Chronic diseases and natural hazards: Impact of disasters on diabetic, renal, and cardiac patients. *Prehosp. Disaster Med.* 2008; 23(02):185–194.

65 Australian Diabetes Educators Association, Diabetes Australia. *The need of people with diabetes and other chronic conditions in natural disasters: A Guide for emergency services, local councils and the not-for-profit sector.* National Diabetes Services Scheme; 2015.

66 Reaves EJ, Termini M, Burkle FM. Reshaping US navy pacific response in mitigating disaster risk in south Pacific Island nations: Adopting community-based disaster cycle management. *Prehosp. Disaster Med.* 2014; 29(1):60–68.

67 Carameli KA, Eisenman DP, Blevins J, d'Angona B, Glik DC. Planning for chronic disease medications in disaster: Perspectives from patients, physicians, pharmacists, and insurers. *Disaster Med. Public Health Prep.* 2013; 7(3):257–265.

68 Arrieta MI, Foreman RD, Crook ED, Icenogle ML. Providing continuity of care for chronic diseases in the aftermath of Katrina: From field experience to policy recommendations. *Disaster Med. Public Health Prep.* 2009; 3(03):174–182.

69 Du W, Little M, Jackson A. Chapter 20: Natural disasters. In: FitzGerald GJ, Tarrant M, Aitken P, Fredriksen M, editors. *Disaster health management: A primer for students and practitioners.* Abingdon, Oxon: Routledge, an imprint of the Taylor & Francis Group; 2017. p. 255–266.

70 Queensland Council of Social Service (QCOSS). APPENDIX 1: Consultation Summary, the Queensland Floods and the Community Sector: Contribution, challenges and lessons for the future. *QCOSS Submission to Floods Inquiry 2011* 2011. http://www.floodcommission.qld.gov.au/__data/assets/file/0008/6983/Qld_Council_of_Social_Service_QCOSS.pdf

71 Kidney Health Australia. *Chronic kidney disease (CKD) management in general practice: Guidance and clinical tips to help identify, manage and refer patients with CKD in your practice.* The Australian Kidney Foundation; 2015.

72 Johnson DW, Hayes B, Gray NA, Hawley C, Hole J, Mantha M. Renal services disaster planning: Lessons learnt from the 2011 queensland floods and north queensland cyclone experiences. *Nephrology* 2013; 18(1):41–46.

73 National Kidney Foundation. *Nutrition and chronic kidney disease (Stages 1-4): Are you getting what you need?* New York, NY: National Kidney Foundation; 2013–14.

74 Ng J, Atkin S, Rigby A, Walton C, Kilpatrick E. The effect of extensive flooding in hull on the glycaemic control of patients with diabetes. *Diabet. Med.* 2011; 28(5):519–524.

75 Mori K, Ugai K, Nonami Y, Kirimura T, Kondo C, Nakamura T, et al. Health needs of patients with chronic diseases who lived through the Great Hanshin Earthquake. *Disaster Manag. Response* 2007; 5(1):8–13.

76 Mudur G. Aid agencies ignored special needs of elderly people after tsunami. *BMJ* 2005; 331(7514):422.

77 Miller-Archie SA, Jordan HT, Ruff RR, Chamany S, Cone JE, Brackbill RM, et al. Posttraumatic stress disorder and new-onset diabetes among adult survivors of the world trade center disaster. *Prev. Med.* 2014; 66:34–38.

78 Irvin CB, Atas JG. Management of evacuee surge from a disaster area: Solutions to avoid non-emergent, emergency department visits. *Prehosp. Disaster Med.* 2007; 22(3):220–223.

79 Thomas VI, Rita G, O'Toole T. A plague on your city: Observations from TOPOFF. *Clin. Infect. Dis.* 2001; 32(3):436–445.

80 Mak PW, Singleton J. Burning questions: Exploring the impact of natural disasters on community pharmacies. *Res. Soc. Admin. Pharm.* 2017; 13(1): 162–171.

# 4 Disaster Theories

## Introduction

In this chapter, we will review the disaster theories that influence and form the decisions made during emergencies. This chapter will be only an overview to give us a basic understanding of the emergency management models used that are relevant to us in the pharmacy profession. Note, we will not be going into depth for each theory or including tangent theories as they are not required to understand how pharmacy can fit within disaster health management. It is important to have an appreciation on how emergency management is typically organised. For example, what readily comes to mind for me is the classic command and control model.

We have covered a lot of the foundational information necessary to understand disasters and emergencies and their impact on our health. So, let's move into the emergency management space of how we actually go about managing and responding to these events. To effectively do this, we need to understand how emergencies are already handled and the theories that are behind the decisions made. It is helpful to understand how decisions are made and the systems at play. For example, this always makes me think of the movies and television shows of emergencies that people love to watch and how there is a strict structure or response procedure that they all follow – person in authority dictates orders and the first responders comply. It is not a coincidence that they all follow this script as this is the most common and historically used theory applied to emergency management.

## Command and Control Theory

The command and control theory is the most utilised in terms of disaster management and has served first responders well for many years and is a pillar of emergency response and war strategies.[1] This theory is centred on the linear and vertical flow of information down the chain of command, with the commander having the authority over the subordinates.[1-3] The military and governments have used command and

DOI: 10.4324/b23292-5

control theory as their standard of management in planning and responding to emergencies and disasters (e.g., the US Marine Corp have indoctrinated this theory into their practice).[1] The rationale for the command and control theory is due to the turbulent environment often found in war and crises situations, orders are able to be given and followed in a rapid, adaptive, and decisive manner.[1] It is suggested command and control theory is necessary for any system, society, or living organism to function.[1]

Some governments and organisations are beginning to see beyond this traditional command and control theory and recognising the value of including community aspects into their emergency management systems.[4,5] This notion of adapting and extending beyond the command and control theory acknowledges that emergencies are becoming more and more complex and presenting uncertain environments which require modifying how operational decisions are made and communicated.[3] To effectively combat these challenging and unknown disaster environments, commanders need timely and accurate information but also need to be flexible to the demands of the situation.[3] By opening up and looking beyond the linear, single flow of communication, it allows for the consideration of the downstream decision consequences, community connections, and communication aspects of emergency and disaster management that have previously been overlooked.[4] The command and control theory is important and still has its place in emergency management, but it is not the sole theory that we should be relying on as it has its limitations.

## Systems Thinking Theory

The looking beyond oneself and considering the consequences of our decisions, lends to the theory of systems thinking. A systems thinking approach allows for a bird's eye view of a problem or issue and allows decision makers to comprehend the potential downstream effects of each potential outcome before implementing changes. It moves away from the traditional, static, analytical problem-solving thought process and takes a more fluid and adaptive, big picture approach.[6] Systems thinking works on the solution to the problem indirectly, focusing upstream of the immediate 'fix' and accounting for all potential outcomes before implementing changes.[6] The fundamental basis of systems thinking is the understanding that there are a multitude of parts that make up any one system, and the system is not just a collection of parts but a functioning unit.[7] To understand a systems thinking approach, we need to understand what is a system and the concept that we live in a – systems of systems.

We as humans are a system and in fact a system made up of systems. We have individual organs that each have a unique purpose and function. An organ on its own is a powerful system that has been specifically engineered to perform. Collectively the human body is made up of more than just the sum total of our organs. So, when we take a medication or eat something, we are not impacting a single isolated organ but impacting the entire body in known and unknown ways. This is true of any system. A system could be seen as a community which is made up of its constituent parts (e.g., people, infrastructure, healthcare, ecosystems, businesses, etc.). For example, governments are a system that consists of several smaller systems (e.g., departments in government, different levels of government, and government as a whole) and each system needs to be adaptable to its ever changing environment.[8]

I love how simply, Dr. Irene Akua Agyepong from the Ministry of Health in Ghana stated in a WHO report on 'Systems Thinking for Health Systems Strengthening' in 2009. She said:

*A systems perspective can minimize the mess; many of today's problems are because of yesterday's solutions.*[6] *(p.51)*

While systems thinking is a complex theory to wrap our heads around, there are two key aspects to systems thinking:

1   Each decision we make has flow-on effects – some that are known/anticipated but some are unknown impacts and consequences. Think of the drug we take that has intended actions and unintended side effects, and
2   A system cannot be broken down into its individual parts. What we mean by this is, the success from a team's effort does not equate to the sum of the contributions made from each individual, as the strength of the team is bigger than just the teammates.[9,10]

Disasters and emergencies are complex and involve many known and unknown risk factors affecting communities and individuals – physically, socially, mentally, economically, and environmentally.[11] If we consider disaster health management there are different systems that are working within this larger system – ambulatory care, tertiary facilities, community support, primary care, search and rescue, etc. Management of emergencies, therefore, requires a holistic approach, as small changes within one system can have drastic flow-on effects downstream in other systems.[12,13]

Currently, emergency management breaks down a disaster into its individual components and each organisation gets given its piece to work on. However, systems thinking suggests disaster and emergency management cannot be broken down into its parts as the 'sum of its parts do not equal the whole system'.[7,14] The key to systems thinking and disaster health management is communication and collaboration between the multitude of organisations providing assistance during and after an emergency.[12,15] Nonetheless, this level of systems thinking collaboration has yet to be achieved, with organisations currently working in disasters operate independently of one another with their own management systems and structures and often overlapping in the services they provide.

If we apply a systems thinking lenses then we would understand and acknowledge that all of our organisations are basically branches all stemming from the same tree, feeding from the same soil. We need to work harmoniously together to achieve the best outcomes for the disaster-affected community, speaking a common language and collectively providing services to those in need. In the context of emergencies and health, a systems thinking approach requires active involvement from the community, and a collaborative relationship between different levels of governments, non-governmental organisations (NGOs), emergency services, healthcare providers, and individuals.[7]

Although taking a systems thinking theory approach will help us to better manage and respond to emergencies, it alone is still not enough to manage complex disasters. Systems thinking is still grounded in the organisational hierarchical leadership and management chain which can often be slow in responding and adapting to emergencies. This has ignited research into the utilisation of chaos theory and its application in emergency management.

## Chaos Theory

Systems thinking and chaos theory are similar in their desire to change the traditional command and control theory to an inclusive model that is capable of fluidity and adaptive change when required. Where these two theories differ however, is that systems thinking is still embedded in the organisational, hierarchical, and formal leadership chain, whereas chaos theory allows for the development of emergent informal leadership unique to the specific crisis.[16,17] Chaos can be a catalyst for change and produce positive emergent behaviour to adequately respond effectively to a disaster or emergency situation. An example of this was the formation of self-coordinated community organisations in response to the 2011 floods in my home state of Queensland, Australia.[18] The community organised what was known in the media as 'Mud Armies'. These were groups of individuals that spontaneously coordinated through social media and armed with shovels and boots helped the clean-up of flood-affected homes.[19,20]

Chaos theory was developed in the 1960s from the work of Edward Lorenz, who identified the higher-order patterns that emerge from what is initially believed to be a chaotic system.[21–23] It is proposed that there is a bifurcation or tipping point within systems which marks the shift where order becomes chaos.[24] For example, the weather is considered chaotic and yet there are patterns in which we can make weather predictions.[22] In this book, we won't be exploring all the learnings of chaos theory as they are beyond what we need to know which is the simplistic notion that 'out of chaos must come order'.

Chaos theory illustrates how systems can develop complex, unpredictably behaviour even though technically its bound by simple rules.[23] This work has further been applied to organisations by Ralph D. Stacey when he introduced the concept of 'The Stacey Matrix'.[23] He explains that in an organisation there are differing levels of agreement between stakeholders and this is dependent upon the level of certainty.[25] Figure 4.1 shows an adapted Stacey Matrix related to emergency management decisions. Simple events are easy to manage as the decision makers can rely on their previous experiences of similar events and group decisions have high consensus.[25] However, complex events are challenging to manage as we cannot rely on previous experiences and there is little agreement among decision makers. So, for disasters that are often complex, unique, unpredictable, and sometimes unrepeatable, we need to approach them differently as our reliance on previous experiences will not be enough.

In understanding the Stacey Matrix, we can see that for simple emergencies like a storm, or a low-grade hurricane, or a small wildfire, the

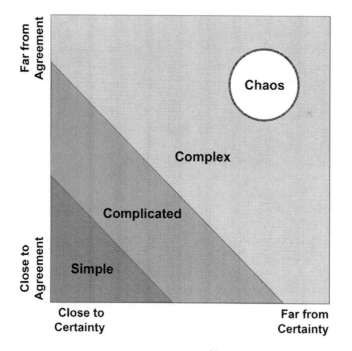

*Figure 4.1* Recreated Stacey Matrix,[23] the further away from agreement and certainty the more complex and chaotic management decisions are for stakeholders.

emergency management decisions and leadership are straight forward and easily agreed upon by the various stakeholders. This is because they rely on their past experiences and the disaster or emergency is contained within their expectations. The problem or challenge lies in when these disaster events become chaotic and there is little agreement between stakeholders regarding management decisions as the event is typically an unpredictable, never-before experienced emergency. Thus, stakeholders cannot rely on their past experiences to make their decisions. Thinking of recent examples – the global COVID-19 pandemic comes readily to mind. There has been widespread disagreement on its management from every corner of the world.

## Surprise Management Theory

Lastly, we will review one more theory that is relevant to how emergency management is structured. A branch or extension of chaos theory that has been applied in emergency management is 'surprise management theory'. It has been suggested by some researchers that surprise management theory is the best approach in incorporating elements of chaos theory and applying it to complex disasters.[24]

Surprise management theory was pioneered by Farazmand and is the theory of managing unknown and complex disasters.[26,27] Surprise management theory consists of four principles and suggests that we need to include other stakeholder's expertise in decision making to adequately manage the chaos of disasters and emergencies.[27] These four principles of surprise management theory are;[27]

1   reject the expected and routine,
2   be flexible, constantly changing and adapting,
3   behaviours consist of a nonlinear and unexplainable relationship which are chaotic or surprising, and
4   expertise and knowledge are essential from stakeholders who are experts in their field, as the skills and attitudes required are beyond the comprehension of those working in the routine environment.

The concept of surprise management theory does not come naturally to many and requires training and resources to be implemented effectively.[26] For example, government departments or administrations do not necessarily have the expertise in managing complex disasters or emergencies and yet they are placed in the position of being required to make decisions regarding emergency management. Surprise management theory suggests that instead of these governments or administrations making the decision based on their best guess or their previous experiences that they actually outsource to experts who understand the chaotic and complexity of disasters and emergency management systems and reject the notion of leaning into their routine response or relying on the ill-fitted expertise of those already within their system.

## Applying These Theories to Pharmacy Practice

So, how do these theories apply to us and our work in disaster pharmacy and disaster health management. We need to acknowledge the importance of each of these theories and when they are appropriate to be used. Command and control theory is a tried-and-true emergency management style that works for simple and localised disasters.[24,26] For example, a hurricane can be a simple disaster – when classed as low grade, directionality can be determined, and because it is a known and experienced emergency. However, hurricanes can also be complex. There is the bifurcation or tipping point that we discussed earlier where the level of management required reaches beyond that of the normal emergency capacity and chaos ensues. For example, Hurricane Katrina.

Disasters are transcending boundaries (i.e., geographical, organisational, etc.) making them complex in their impact on the communities, the organisations involved, and in the response required.[9,28,29] Natural hazards are not only increasing with frequency and intensity but are impacting communities with unprecedented force,[9] suggesting even simple localised emergencies are being underestimated for their associated disaster risks. The question that is posed for us is, 'When does a disaster go beyond the bifurcation or tipping point and become complex enough to require a mixed theory approach over a simple command and control method?'

Let's look at an example specific to pharmacy from the recent global COVID-19 pandemic. I think we can all agree that the COVID-19 pandemic presents a complex disaster challenge. In the early phase of the pandemic, many parts of the world were experiencing medication shortages. In an effort to address this, governments brought in temporary rules limiting or rationing the supply of medications in North America. So, patients that typically would receive 100-day supply of medications were now getting 30-day supplies. This sounds like a smart, practical decision and strategy to reduce the impact of the international medication shortages and ensure equitable access to all. While this may still have been the case, this simple linear approach to the problem did not consider the downstream effects of such a decision. The reduction in supply was temporary and as the supply chain began to stabilise again, the ruling was revoked, and the 100-day supply of medications was reinstated. Problem solved, right? Not quite. Because once the supply was reverted back to 100-day supply, pharmacies were now faced with the challenge of all of their patients being due for their large quantities of 100-day supplies of medications at the exact same time and it repeats in a cycle every 100 days. So, every 100 days, the workload of pharmacies drastically increases, and there is this 'boom and bust' impact on their inventory.

In healthcare and emergency management, we have to consider the full picture and try to understand some of the known consequences and challenges that will result from the decisions we make. It won't be perfect as there will be unknown impacts that we might not be able to predict but that is why we practice and participate in preparedness activities to workshop these decisions before emergencies happen with other stakeholders in a safe learning environment. This helps us see emergency management with a systems thinking and surprise management mindset.

## Chapter References

1  U.S. Marine Corps. *MCDP 6 command and control. Department of the Navy.* Wasington D.C.: Marine Corp Doctrinal Publications; 1996.

2  Chaudhury K, Nibedita A, Mishra P. Command and control in disaster management. *International Journal of Computer Science Issues (IJCSI)* 2012; 9(4):256–259.

3  Rosen J, Grigg E, Lanier J, McGrath S, Lillibridge S, Sargent D, et al. The future of command and control for disaster response. *IEEE Eng. Med. Biol. Mag.* 2002; 21(5):56–68.

4  Emergency Management VictoriaThe six C's [Internet]. Melbourne, Victoria: State of Victoria; 2018 [cited 2019 3rd Feb]; Available from: http://www.webcitation.org/75tbVKyJ1

5  Lapsley C, Ferguson E, Goodwin A, Rau P, White T. *Fundamentals of emergency management (Class 1 emergencies) edition 1. Department of Justice and Regulation.* Melbourne, Victoria: Emergency Management Victoria, Victorian Government; 2015.

6  De Savigny D, Adam T. *Systems thinking for health systems strengthening.* Geneva, Switzerland: World Health Organization; 2009. p. 1–112.

7  Cavallo A. Integrating disaster preparedness and resilience: A complex approach using system of systems. *Australian Journal of Emergency Management* 2014; 29(3):46–51.

8  Checkland P. Systems thinking. In: Currie W, Galliers B, editors. *Rethinking management information systems an interdisciplinary perspective.* Oxford: OUP Oxford; 1999.

9  Cavallo A, Ireland V. Preparing for complex interdependent risks: A system of systems approach to building disaster resilience. *Inter. J. Dis. Risk Red.* 2014; 9:181–193.

10  Checkland P. Systems thinking and soft systems methodology. In: Galliers RD, Currie WL, editors. *The Oxford handbook of management information systems: Critical perspectives and new directions.* Oxford University Press; 2011. vol 1.

11  International Strategy for Disaster Reduction (ISDR), United Nations. Hyogo Framework for Action 2005–2015: Building the Resilience of Nations and Communities to Disasters. In: Extract from the final report of the World Conference on Disaster Reduction (A/CONF. 206/6); 2005.

12 Leischow SJ, Best A, Trochim WM, Clark PI, Gallagher RS, Marcus SE, et al. Systems thinking to improve the public's health. *Am. J. Prev. Med.* 2008; 35(2):S196–S203.

13 Fawcett AM, Fawcett SE. Benchmarking the state of humanitarian aid and disaster relief: A systems design perspective and research agenda. *Benchmarking* 2013; 20(5):661–692.

14 Cavallo A, Ireland V. SoS in disasters: Why following the manual can be a mistake. In: System of systems engineering (SoSE), 2012 7th International Conference IEEE; 2012. p. 161–166.

15 Palttala P, Boano C, Lund R, Vos M. Communication gaps in disaster management: Perceptions by experts from governmental and non-governmental organizations. *J. Contingencies Crisis Manag.* 2012; 20(1):2–12.

16 Uhl-Bien M, Marion R, McKelvey B. Complexity leadership theory: Shifting leadership from the industrial age to the knowledge era. *Leadersh Q* 2007; 18(4):298–318.

17 Osborn RN, Hunt JG. Leadership and the choice of order: Complexity and hierarchical perspectives near the edge of chaos. *Leadersh Q* 2007; 18(4):319–340.

18 Morris Jr GW. *The chaos of Katrina.* Air Force Institute of Technology; 2007:104.

19 Rafter F. Volunteers as agents of co-production: 'Mud armies' in emergency services. In: *Putting citizens first: Engagement in policy and service delivery for the 21st century.* Canberra: ANU E Press: The Australian National University; 2013. p. 187–192.

20 Hartel CEJ, Latemore GM. Mud and tears: The human face of disaster – A case study of the Queensland Floods, January 2011. *Journal Of Management and Organisation* 2011; 17(6):864–872.

21 Lorenz EN. Deterministic nonperiodic flow. *J. Atmos. Sci.* 1963; 20(2):130–141.

22 Gleick J. *Chaos: Making a new science.* London: Cardinal; 1988.

23 Stacey RD. *Complexity and creativity in organizations.* Berrett-Koehler Publishers; 1996.

24 Koehler GA, Kress GG, Miller RL. What disaster response management can learn from chaos theory. In: *Crisis and emergency management: Theory and practice* 2014; 178:111–130.

25 Zimmerman B. Ralph Stacey's agreement & certainty matrix [Internet]. Edgeware – Aides,2001 [cited 2016 31st October]; Available from: http://www.webcitation.org/6lfM7b9Xb

26 Farazmand A. Hurricane Katrina, the crisis of leadership, and chaos management: Time for trying the 'surprise management theory in action'. *Pub. Org. Rev.* 2009; 9(4):399–412.

27 Farazmand A. Learning from the Katrina crisis: A global and international perspective with implications for future crisis management. *Pub. Adm. Rev.* 2007; 67:149–159.

28 McGuire, B. (Global Disaster Paves Way for Global Thinking: In the Wake of the Indian Ocean Tsunami, Disaster Expert and Geophysicist Bill Mcguire Explains why Future Disaster Management Must Place a Greater Emphasis on Preparedness as well as Response. *Geographical.* 2005; 77(3):14.

29 Leischow, SJ, & Milstein, B. Systems Thinking and Modeling for Public Health Practice. *Am. J. Public Health.* 2006; 96(3):403–405.

# 5 Disaster and Emergency Pharmacy Models

## Introduction

We have discussed in the previous chapters the foundational understanding of disasters and emergency management. Now that we have this background, let's hone into the specific field of interest for all of us – that of disaster pharmacy. If you haven't read the previous chapters yet, I would encourage you to go back and read them. It's important to understand the larger picture of where disaster pharmacy fits within the greater context of emergency management and disaster health.

This is a relevantly new field of study and there have been some that have paved the way and attempted to synthesis and categorise pharmacists' roles during emergencies. There are different ways to view or frame pharmacists' positions, roles, and services in disasters. We are going to review the existing disaster and emergency pharmacy models together, and then I will present the model I developed with consensus from an international expert panel.

## Role Categorisation Model

In 2004, a model of pharmacists' roles during bioterrorism events was suggested by Dr Paul Setlak in a commentary published in the American Journal of Health-System Pharmacy. Dr Setlak listed potential roles that health-system pharmacists in the US could fulfil during bioterrorism emergencies and separated these roles into four categories.[1] These categories are:[1–3]

- **Response integration** – Response integration refers to a first responder role for pharmacists and assisting in areas where there are shortages of healthcare professionals.
- **Patient management** – Patient management refers to pharmacist roles in providing patient management in the aftermath of an emergency
- **Pharmaceutical supply** – Pharmaceutical supply falls within the traditional role of pharmacists focusing on the procurement and logistics

DOI: 10.4324/b23292-6

- *Policy coordination* – Policy coordination refers to the role pharmacists can play in assisting the development of guidance, algorithms, and patient assessment tools used in the rapid dispersal of prophylaxis treatment following bioterrorism threats

This role categorisation model developed by Dr Setlak has been extended by another US research – Dr Heath Ford, to also apply to natural hazards.[2,3] However, this role categorisation model is theoretical and was not originally designed or developed to include an all-hazard approach to emergencies. Additionally it was specifically designed for health-system pharmacists, which in the United States is predominately hospital-based practice.

## Disaster Readiness Model

In 2011, another model was proposed by Dr. Laura Pincock and colleagues. Their disaster readiness model was suggested in another commentary published in the American Journal of Health-System Pharmacy.[4] This model categorised pharmacists' roles for emergencies based on the pharmacist's practice setting (ambulatory care, pharmacotherapy and critical care, logistics, pandemics/weapons of mass destruction, and management). Pharmacists' roles in emergencies were divided into two categories – clinical and other. The clinical category covered roles involving direct patient care, medication management, and ambulatory care roles. The other category included specialised and non-clinical roles (e.g., logistics, management, etc.). However, this model also has limitations, as it makes the assumption that pharmacists only work in those specific environments and that they are mutually exclusive.

## Pharmacy Personnel Model

In 2016, the International Pharmacy Federation (FIP) published guidelines for the roles of pharmacy personnel and was categorised by their practice setting (e.g., hospital, community, government, and industry).[5] They outline that government, pharmacy industry, and pharmacy associations have the responsibility to perform the risk analysis for the pharmacy profession in terms of emergency management.[5] Unsurprisingly, they suggest it is the government pharmacy's role to advocate and implement the amendment to legislation allowing for expanded scope for pharmacist roles in disasters and emergencies. For hospital and community pharmacies, they recommend they perform their own risk analysis and practice emergency drills following emergency protocols. Additionally, hospital pharmacy personnel should advocate and implement any amended legislation to expand pharmacy's duties, maintain records, and coordinate supply of pharmaceuticals. FIP also suggests for community pharmacies to maintain health records, implement amended legislations, and managing the resources (both human and pharmaceuticals).[5] Following a disaster or emergency, hospital and community pharmacy personnel should participate in post-disaster after-action reports reflecting on lessons learned.[5]

Similarly in 2017, a model was proposed by Dr. Alkhalili and colleagues in a literature review.[6] Their model was developed by matching pharmacists' roles and core competencies to the differing levels of qualifications of pharmacy personnel. They acknowledged that the roles of pharmacy personnel change over the course of an emergency and depending on the different levels of competency and qualifications of the pharmacy personnel available to respond to the emergency. To determine the key activities required in an emergency, they developed five core capabilities which pharmacy personnel should strive to achieve and maintain in an emergency. The pharmacy personnel identified in this study were pharmacy technicians, pharmacists, and an additional level of competency for pharmacy managers and specialist pharmacists (advanced scope pharmacists) within the pharmacy profession.[6] These capabilities were described as:[6]

- *Professional practice* – The professional practice capability entails pharmacy taking a leadership role and ensures the pharmacy remains operational or returns to operational as quickly as possible following an emergency.
- *Population health planning* – The population health planning capability involves being aware of the health of the community in which the pharmacy is located, developing risk mitigation plans to improve the health of the community, and developing plans for how the pharmacy will run in the event of an emergency.
- *Direct patient care* – The direct patient care capability involves developing coordinated individual care plans and continuing medication management services.
- *Legislation* – The legislation capability refers to understand the current legislation in place for the region and advocate for amendments to utilise pharmacist's full scope of practice.
- *Communications* – The communications capability involves maintaining communication channels and record keeping.

## Challenges with Existing Models

There are different ways to view or frame pharmacists' positions in disasters. All these models we have discussed set out the tasks, actions, or core competencies for pharmacists and pharmacy personnel during emergencies and provide a great starting point for identifying pharmacists' roles in disasters. However, they are needed collectively to understand the scope, breadth, and responsibilities of pharmacists during emergencies. For example, some of them do not consider pharmacists as a clinical healthcare professional that can move beyond the 'bricks and mortar' workplace context of pharmacies.

So, I propose in this chapter a different categorisation model that builds on the foundations provided by these other researchers but also uses categories that are commonly understood and recognised by the wider emergency management field. The model I am proposing in this book was conceptually developed from a mixed methods study I conducted that included surveys, interviews, and a Delphi Study to obtain consensus from international experts on pharmacists' roles during emergencies and I specifically used an all-hazard approach.[7] To remind you, an all-hazard approach allows for the development of a single disaster and emergency management plan and strategies to account for any conceivable hazard, unknowns, and their mutual relationships to each other.[8] In this context, what are the pharmacists' roles for any and all types of emergencies? This model consists of two parts:

1   *Where do pharmacists fit* – Conceptualising pharmacists' roles in the overarching emergency management categories as presented in this chapter using the identified four practice area categories – logistics, public health, patient care, and governance,[9,10] and
2   *PPRR cycle and pharmacist roles* – In Chapter 7, we will delve deeper into each of these categories and discuss specific pharmacists' roles and services as they span across the PPRR cycle of emergency management.

It is important to remember that the roles and responsibilities pharmacists might be required to fulfil during an emergency all depend on where the emergency occurs, what healthcare services have been affected, and what healthcare resources and professionals are available to assist. What we will focus on in this Chapter is understanding the four broad practice areas in which these roles can be categorised.

## Where Do Pharmacists Fit: A Disaster Pharmacy Model

### Introduction

Emergency management has many subsections with four of the bigger ones being – logistics, governance, patient care, and public health. However, often each of these subsections are 'siloed' or managed mutually exclusive to each other. This poses a challenge for us in the pharmacy profession. Because we contribute to all four subsections in everyday practice,[11-15] but when it comes to emergencies pharmacists are often pigeon-holed into their tried-and-true traditional role of medication logistics. This limits our ability to make substantial contributions to the other subsections within our scope of practice and expertise. Logistics and medicine supply is an extremely important pharmacist role and should not be dismissed or underestimated, but it is simply not the only tool at the disposal of pharmacists.

This pigeon-holing does not make a lot of sense, as during a crisis there are often shortages in resources and healthcare professionals. So, boxing pharmacists out of using their full scope of practice does a disservice to patients and disaster-affected individuals. We need to operate at a systems thinking level, sharing resources and services amongst the healthcare system and to carry the interprofessional and collaborative nature of healthcare into emergency situations. Pharmacists need to be accepted and acknowledged for their ability to bring a unique skillset and knowledge to disaster management and be allowed to transcend the boundaries of the restrictive individual practice areas.

The term practice areas, I am using in this model does not refer to a specific position or employment context for a pharmacist but is referencing a way to conceptualise the vast roles and services pharmacists provide in overarching categories that relate to the emergency management field. Figure 5.1 illustrates the key aspects of these four practice areas. So, let's look at each practice area in more detail.

### Logistics

When we mention the concept of drugs in emergency management, people call on pharmacists. But often this is too late and misses valuable

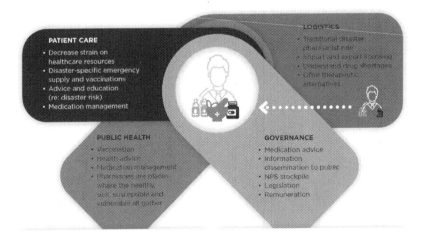

*Figure 5.1* Conceptual framework model of pharmacists' current logistics practice area and how they should be allowed to transcend the boundaries into multiple practice areas. *Figure developed by author and illustrated by Bushfire and Natural Hazard CRC, reproduced with permission.*[9]

insight from the pharmacists on relevant health decisions. Additionally, when the concept or immediate need for drugs goes away so too does the seeking of input from pharmacists. However, this is short-sighted as pharmacists bring a unique understanding of medicines to the role of logistics that is important during the preparedness phase as well as the response.

Pharmacists and logisticians are different, and pharmacists bring their clinical knowledge with them to these positions which is invaluable. For example, you are in a field hospital setting following an earthquake and there are challenges with getting cephalexin antibiotic stock which is needed for several patients. Typically the logistician will inform you that they do not have any stock and ask you if could you use something else. Whereas the pharmacist may say we don't have any cephalexin stock available but I did a review and for this patient trimethoprim would also work and here is the rationale of why I recommend that. Pharmacists are able to bring their clinical knowledge and expertise to the role of logistics and it goes beyond simply getting things from A to B.

Pharmacists professionally straddle multiple entities including both the logistics and the medical fields, speaking both languages but not fully belonging to either. The role of pharmacists in ensuring medications are available in emergencies throughout the different stages of the logistics supply chain is essential.[16] NGOs working in emergencies and humanitarian crises have developed complex systems in which to access maintainable medication supplies and they often utilise the expertise of pharmacists.[16]

### Public Health

Pharmacists work across both the medical and public health sectors looking after the welfare of patients and the community in everyday circumstances and in times of disasters. This has become even more apparent recently as the mass media has focused on pharmacists' contributions during the COVID-19 pandemic. It is known that patients avoid aspects of the healthcare system during emergencies out of fear, anxiety, or expected long wait times. These patients seek out pharmacies due to their accessibility and their anchoring place within the community.[17,18] Dr. Fredrick (Skip) Burkle Jr mentioned in his interview (the full interview is available in Chapter 8) that disasters and emergencies quickly become public health crises and therefore all healthcare practitioners need to have public health skills and knowledge to confidently undertake their roles and responsibilities. This includes pharmacists and pharmacy personnel.

In terms of pharmacy, the concept of public health is encompassed with the mandate of equitable access to medicines. Pharmacists in everyday practice undertake several key roles within the public health domain (e.g., patient safety, pharmacovigilance, harm minimisation, rational drug use, vaccination programs, prevention campaigns, contraception services, and emergency management).[12,19] These become even more important during an emergency with the loss of existing public health infrastructure and the additional pressures placed on the healthcare system.

### Patient Care

It has been well documented that pharmacists' involvement in patient care leads to improved patient safety and outcomes. A systematic review conducted in 2010 found that including pharmacists as team members in the provision of direct patient care improved various patient outcomes (such as reduced adverse drug events and improved patient education) across different disease states and in different healthcare settings.[14] This has also extended to pharmacists' involvement in emergencies. The Thunderstorm Asthma event in 2016 in Australia resulted in an after-action report being completed by the Australian Victorian state government Inspector General Emergency Management office and they acknowledged that without pharmacists involvement the mortality rate could have been much higher and suggested that pharmacists should be included on health teams to improve outcomes in emergencies.[20] We will look at this event in more detail in Chapter 6.

It is known that most patients when displaced or evacuated leave without their medications or prescriptions.[21] Who else apart from pharmacy is better positioned to meet these needs and reduce the burden on the healthcare system for ambulatory and low-acuity patients. By giving pharmacists more authority in disasters to adequately look after the needs of patients with chronic conditions, doctors and nurses can focus their attention and resources on more critically ill patients.[22] This has been the case historically, in improving hospital systems and reducing the number of medication errors.[23] One such study found that over the span of four months in 2007 in a single hospital in Detroit, United States, pharmacists working in the ED saved the healthcare system over $1 billion in cost avoidance interventions.[24] By extension, with the surge capacity expected during an emergency in a hospital ED, including pharmacists would potentially increase this cost saving exponentially. However, we need more documented evidence of how pharmacist-led initiatives are cost saving measures to the healthcare system and improve patient outcomes.

### Governance

It is suggested that governments and health departments tend to have a narrow view on healthcare services and the professionals necessary to provide them, often overlooking community services (e.g., pharmacies, family physicians' clinics, etc.) or the private sector and focusing on emergency services and government funded hospitals.

I strongly suggest and advocate that pharmacists need to be more proactive in the governance space. Pharmacists and pharmacy organisations need to advocate for representation of pharmacy at the national, subnational, and local levels for health policy decisions and especially in emergency management. It needs to be understood by our governments how pharmacy legislation can enable or hinder pharmacists' ability to assist in an emergency and the operational challenges of the decisions they make during emergency response.[25]

How will our governments know what is happening on the frontline if we don't tell them? A classic example that came out of the COVID-19 pandemic, was the ever-changing rules for eligibility for COVID vaccines. Pharmacists and their staff around the world were single-handedly providing the vast majority of these mass vaccinations in addition to their other daily tasks and COVID-19 specific roles. Yet, every time there was a change in the eligibility, a government official would make a public announcement in the media before communicating the change to the pharmacists administering this service. So, pharmacists in the middle of their workday were being inundated with phone calls and people flocking to their pharmacies with questions and asking for their vaccines. Did the government think that the pharmacists were listening into the public announcement while in the middle of their workday activities? By not having effective communication channels established, pharmacists and their staff were not able to appropriately respond by increasing their staffing requirements or putting measures in place to cope with the new rules. This may have been a simple oversight but then it continued two years into the ongoing pandemic. To me it seems disrespectful and undervaluing the profession that we have relied on so heavily to get us through this public health crisis. I wonder where are the pharmacy lobby groups, advocacy, or professional organisations representing the frontline at the government level? But also, is it their sole responsibility? Pharmacists were complaining about the lack of communication but who were they complaining to – only each other? We all need to take our responsibility of advocacy and governance seriously as it is vital in effective emergency management.

## Chapter References

1 Setlak P. Bioterrorism preparedness and response: Emerging role for health-system pharmacists. *Am. J. Health Syst. Pharm.* 2004; 61(11):1167–1175.

2 Ford JH. *Pharmacists in disasters* [PhD Thesis]. Athens, Gerogia: University of Georgia; 2013.

3 Ford H, Dallas CE, Harris C. Examining roles pharmacists assume in disasters: A content analytic approach. *Dis. Med. Public Health Prep.* 2013; 7(06):563–572.

4 Pincock LL, Montello MJ, Tarosky MJ, Pierce WF, Edwards CW. Pharmacist readiness roles for emergency preparedness. *Am. J. Health Syst. Pharm.* 2011; 68(7):620.

5 International Pharmaceutical Federation (FIP). *Responding to disasters: Guidelines for pharmacy 2016.* The Hague: International Pharmaceutical Federation; 2016.

6 Alkhalili M, Ma J, Grenier S. Defining roles for pharmacy personnel in disaster response and emergency preparedness. *Dis. Med. Public Health Prep.* 2017; 11(4):1–9.

7 Watson KE. *The roles of pharmacists in disaster health management in natural and anthropogenic disasters.* [Thesis]. QUT ePrints: Queensland University of Technology; 2019 Available from: https://eprints.qut.edu.au/130757/

8 Lettieri E, Masella C, Radaelli G. Disaster management: Findings from a systematic review. *Dis. Prevent. Manage.* 2009; 18(2):117–136.

9 Watson KE. *Hazard Note 78: On the frontline: The roles of pharmacists in disasters.* Bushfire and Natural Hazard CRC; 2020.

10 Watson KE. *An unassuming pair: Pharmacists and disasters. Asia Pacific Fire Magazine*; 2021.

11 Bruce Bayley K, Savitz LA, Maddalone T, Stoner SE, Hunt JS, Wells R. Evaluation of patient care interventions and recommendations by a transitional care pharmacist. *Ther. Clin. Risk Manag.* 2007; 3(4):695–703.

12 Jackson JK, Snell B, Sweidan M, Duncan G, Spinks J. Public health-recognising the role of Australian pharmacists. *J. Phar. Prac. Res.* 2004; 34(4):290–292.

13 Patwardhan A, Duncan I, Murphy P, Pegus C. The value of pharmacists in health care. *Popul. Health Manag.* 2012; 15(3):157–162.

14 Chisholm-Burns MA, Lee JK, Spivey CA, Slack M, Herrier RN, Hall-Lipsy E, et al. US pharmacists' effect as team members on patient care: Systematic review and meta-analyses. *Med. Care* 2010; 48(10):923–933.

15 Paolini N, Rouse MJ. Scope of contemporary pharmacy practice: Roles, responsibilities, and functions of pharmacists and pharmacy technicians executive summary. *Am. J. Health Syst. Pharm.* 2010; 67(12):1030–1031.

16 Villacorta-Linaza R. Bridging the gap: The role of pharmacists in managing the drug supply cycle within non-governmental organizations. *Int. J. Health Plann. Manage.* 2009; 24(S1):S73–S86.

17 Ford H, Trent S, Wickizer S. Pharmacy services after a tank car derailment and toxic chemical release in Blount County, Tennessee. *J. Am. Pharm. Assoc.* (2003) 2017; 57(1):56–61.e2.

18 Austin Z, Martin JC, Gregory PA. Pharmacy practice in times of civil crisis: The experience of SARs and "the blackout" in Ontario, Canada. *Res. Soc. Admin. Phar.* 2007; 3(3):320–335.

19 Stergachis A, Lander RD, Webb LE. Promoting the pharmacist's role in public health. *J. Am. Pharm. Assoc.* (2003) 2006; 46(3):311–319.

20 Inspector-General for Emergency Management (IGEM), Victorian Government. Review of response to the thunderstorm asthma event of 21–22 November 2016: Final report. 2017.

21 Ochi SHS, Landeg O, Mayner L, Murray V. Disaster-driven evacuation and medication loss: A systematic literature review. *PLoS Curr. Dis.* 2014; 18(6):1–20.

22 Lai E, Trac L, Lovett A. Expanding the pharmacist's role in public health. *Univers. J. Pub. Heal.* 2013; 1(3):79–85.

23 Leape LL. Errors in medicine. *Clin. Chim. Acta* 2009; 404(1):2–5.

24 Lada P, Delgado G. Documentation of pharmacists' interventions in an emergency department and associated cost avoidance. *Am. J. Health Syst. Pharm.* 2007; 64(1):63–68.

25 Watson, KE, Singleton, JA, Tippett, V, Nissen, LM. Do disasters predict international pharmacy legislation? *Aust Health Rev.* 2019; 44:392–398.

# Part II

# Pharmacists' Place in Disaster and Emergency Management

# 6 The History and Evolution of Pharmacists in Disasters and Emergencies

## Introduction

This section of the book has me really excited as I think it's important for us to recognise the progress that pharmacists have already made in emergency management and to be aware of those that came before. Maybe, we can even learn from their challenges and mistakes. In this chapter we will take a walk down memory lane together and review the history and evolution of pharmacists' roles in disasters and emergencies. You will see that there have been some significant events that have occurred in various regions that have propelled pharmacists' roles and services forward. We will also take a specific look at the COVID-19 pandemic, being the most recent and heavily studied emergency event to-date.

I must preface this chapter with a note of caution that this is not an extensive history and there may be gaps. I am not a historian and have compiled all the recorded major events that I could find within the published literature. Fortunately for us, there was a historian or two that took an interest in this topic and documented some of pharmacists' roles and services from as early as the American Civil War,[1] the World Wars,[2] and the Spanish flu pandemic.[3] Many of these documented accounts are from the United States, this doesn't mean pharmacists weren't involved in emergencies elsewhere in the world or other emergency events but that it has not been recorded in available published literature.

## History of Pharmacists in Emergencies

There have been some key major disaster and emergency events throughout history that have significantly propelled pharmacists' roles in emergency management forward. But this story is not over, there is plenty of room for the pharmacy profession to grow in disaster and emergency management and ... the next chapters of history have yet to be written by us. I love this quote written by Scott and Constantine in 1990, that recognises how valuable pharmacists always have been in our communities and why we are important in emergency management.

DOI: 10.4324/b23292-8

*… everyone in the community depends on the pharmacists to be among the first to recover.*[4]

### Major Disasters and Emergencies

Table 6.1 outlines some of the published literature and documents regarding pharmacists' roles and services during previous disaster and emergency events. What is interesting to note is that over 70% of the articles listed were about events that occurred within the United States. The United States has faced some significant events that have shaped and propelled pharmacists' roles in emergency management forward, with pharmacists recognised as clinical and essential members of their Disaster Medical Assistance Teams (DMATs). This does not discredit the work frontline pharmacists have contributed to in disaster and emergency events in other regions, as it is commonly understood that pharmacists step up and meet the needs of any presenting emergency within their communities. But it does highlight where the current documented research and understanding of pharmacists' roles in emergencies is centred and identifies the overwhelming gap and need for more documented evidence of the pivotal roles and services pharmacists provide in other regions.

Important pharmacists' roles and services in emergencies can be hard to categorise as put simply, pharmacists meet the needs of the disaster-affected community and individuals. This encompasses anything and everything from calming fears and anxiety, explaining public health measures, providing medications, providing general necessities and supplies, coordinating logistics for inventory management, prescribing, triaging, screening, outreach, being accessible and many more roles. So what I have tried to achieve in Table 6.1 is an outline of research articles about specific emergency events and highlighted the main pharmacists' roles described in each article.

### American Civil War

The earliest published report that I could source that mentioned the role of pharmacists in disasters, emergencies, and conflicts was a book written by a historian named Michael Flannery. He wrote a book titled *Civil War pharmacy: A history of drugs, drug supply and provision, and therapeutics for the Union and Confederacy.*[1] In his book, he describes how the civil war that began in 1861 played a significant role in shaping the healthcare industry in the United States as it stands today. During the war these medical and health fields were in their infancy or non-existent. The medical profession became organised in 1847 with the founding of the American Medical Association and pharmacists established their own American Pharmaceutical Association a few years

*Table 6.1* List of some of published literature regarding pharmacists' roles and services during previous disaster events up until 2019

| Authors | Country | Major Event | Main Pharmacists' Roles |
|---|---|---|---|
| MacCara ME. [3] | Canada | 1918 Spanish Flu Pandemic | Medication management<br>Compounding |
| Grabenstein JD. [5] | US | 1984 Oregon salmonella intentional poisoning | Information resource |
| Cramer R, Weeks K. [6] | US | 1989 Alabama tornado | Inventory management<br>Medication management |
| Scott S, Constantine LM. [4] | US | 1989 Hurricane Hugo, a California earthquake, and a Colorado Tornado | Meeting the needs of the disaster-affected individuals<br>Coping with power outages<br>Securing narcotics |
| Carda E, Harcum J, Olthoff C. [7] | US | 1989 Iowa plane crash | Triage<br>Information resource<br>Temporary pharmacy set-up and services<br>Inventory management |
| Nestor A, Aviles AI, Kummerle DR, et al. [8] | US | 1992 Hurricane Andrew | Temporary pharmacy set-up and services<br>Manage donated medicines<br>Information resource |
| Merges V. [9] | US | 1992 Hurricane Iniki | Inventory management |
| Miller C. [10] | US | 1992 Hurricane Iniki | Temporary pharmacy set-up and services<br>Inventory management<br>Medication management |
| Bussières J-F, St-Arnaud C, Schunck C, et al. [11] | Bosnia-Herzegovina | 1992–1999 Bosni-Herzegovina conflict and humanitarian relief | Inventory management<br>Manage donated medicines |

(Continued)

*Table 6.1* (Continued)

| Authors | Country | Major Event | Main Pharmacists' Roles |
|---|---|---|---|
| Lambert E.[12] | Senegal | Casamance conflict | Manage donated medicines<br>Train health workers |
| Bethea S.[13] | US | 1993 Train derailed mobile | Medication management<br>Information resource<br>Inventory management |
| Leduc D, Levy D.[14] | US | 1994 Northridge earthquake | Temporary pharmacy set-up and services<br>Information resource<br>Medication management<br>Clinical DMAT member |
| Sagraves R.[15] | US | 1995 Oklahoma City Bombing | Inventory management |
| Burda AM, Sigg T.[16] | Japan | 1995 Sarin Tokyo Subway attack, | Information resource |
|  | US | 2001 Anthrax crisis | Inventory management |
| Berod T, Chan-ou-Teung F.[17] | French Island, Indian Ocean | 1996 Plane crash | Inventory management<br>Meeting the needs of the disaster-affected individuals |
| Montello MJ, Ostroff C, Frank EC, et al.[18] | US | 2001 Anthrax crisis | Prophylaxis management<br>Information resource<br>Screening |
| Haffer AS, James R R, Montello MJ, et al.[19] | US | 2001 Anthrax crisis | Prophylaxis management<br>Information resource<br>Prescribing |
| Babb J, Downs K.[20] | US | 2001 September 11 terrorist attacks | Inventory management |
| Gaudette R, Schnitzer J, George E, Briggs SM.[21] | US | 2001 September 11 terrorist attacks | First responder<br>Clinical DMAT member |

| Reference | Country | Event | Roles |
|---|---|---|---|
| Babb J, Tosatto R, Hayslett J.[22] | US | 2001 September 11 terrorist attacks, Anthrax crisis | Prophylaxis management; Information resource |
| Cohen V.[23] | US | 2001 September 11 terrorist attacks, Anthrax crisis | Information resource; Inventory management; Pharmacy emergency response team (PERT) member |
| Chin TWF, Chant C, Tanzini R, Wells J.[24] | Canada | 2003 SARS outbreak | Information resource; Train health workers |
| Austin Z, Martin JC, Gregory PA.[25] | Canada | 2003 severe acute respiratory syndrome (SARS) outbreak | First responder; Information resource |
| Mason P.[26] | Indonesia | 2004 Boxing day tsunami | Manage donated medicines |
| Kirtley JC.[27] | US | 2005 Gulf Coast hurricanes | Temporary pharmacy set-up and services |
| Lynas K.[28] | US | 2005 Hurricane Katrina | Triage; Temporary pharmacy set-up and services; Medication management |
| Velazquez L, Dallas S, Rose L, et al.[29] | US | 2005 Hurricane Katrina | Temporary pharmacy set-up and services |
| Russum M.[30] | US | 2005 Hurricane Katrina | Medication management; Temporary pharmacy set-up and services |
| Henderson GS.[31] | US | 2005 Hurricane Katrina | Inventory management |
| Geraci SA, Douglas S, Algood TL, et al.[32] | US | 2005 Hurricane Katrina | Medication management; Temporary pharmacy set-up and services |
| Kaldy J.[33] | US | 2005 Hurricane Katrina | Medication management |
| Young D.[34] | US | 2005 Hurricane Katrina | Clinical DMAT member |

*(Continued)*

*Table 6.1* (Continued)

| Authors | Country | Major Event | Main Pharmacists' Roles |
|---|---|---|---|
| Bratberg J.[35] | US | 2005 Hurricane Katrina | Temporary pharmacy set-up and services<br>Medication management<br>Meeting the needs of the disaster-affected individuals<br>Clinical DMAT member |
| Bethea S.[36] | US | 2005 Hurricane Katrina | Temporary pharmacy set-up and services<br>Information resource<br>Inventory management |
| Hogue MD, Hogue HB, Lander RD, Avent K, Fleenor M.[37] | US | 2005 Hurricane Katrina | Triage<br>Screening<br>Prescribing<br>Temporary pharmacy set-up and services<br>Information resource |
| Jhung MA, Shehab N, Rohr-Allegrini C, et al.[38] | US | 2005 Hurricane Katrina | Medication management |
| Lust E.[39] | US | 2005 Hurricane Katrina | Triage<br>Temporary pharmacy set-up and services<br>Information resource<br>Manage donated medicines<br>Clinical member of veterinary Medical assistance teams |
| Labdi BA.[40] | US | 2005 Hurricane Rita | Inventory management<br>Discharge patients<br>Clinical emergency team members |
| Gershgol SM, Cantrell L, Mutrux B.[41] | US | 2007 California wildfires | Using pharmacy students to backfill pharmacist roles and increase capacity of pharmacy services |

| Author | Event | Country | Roles |
|---|---|---|---|
| Bhavsar TR, Kim H-J, Yu Y.[42] | 2009 H1N1 pandemic | US | Prophylaxis management<br>Information resource<br>Screening |
| Schwerzmann J, Graitcer SB, Jester B, Krahl D, et al.[43] | 2009 H1N1 pandemic | US | Administer vaccinations |
| Huynh C, Lott A.[44] | 2010 Haiti earthquake | Haiti | Meeting the needs of the disaster-affected individuals |
| Ferris D.[45] | 2010 Haiti earthquake | Haiti | Medication management |
| Hashimoto T, Sato H.[46] | 2011 Great East Japan Earthquake | Japan | Temporary pharmacy set-up and services |
| Takeda Y.[47] | 2011 Great East Japan Earthquake | Japan | First responder<br>Clinical DMAT member<br>Using pharmacy students to backfill pharmacist roles<br>Temporary pharmacy set-up and services<br>Manage donated medicines |
| Kawataba Y.[48] | 2011 Great East Japan Earthquake | Japan | Inventory management<br>Medication Management |
| Epp DA, Tanno Y, Brown A, Brown B.[49] | 2011 Great East Japan Earthquake, 2013 Calgary flood | Japan/Canada | Temporary pharmacy set-up and services<br>Information resource<br>Prescribing |
| Mak PW, Singleton J.[50] | 2012–2013 Tasmanian bushfires | Australia | Inventory management |
| Erickson K.[51] | 2013 Boston marathon bombing | US | Discharge patients<br>Triage<br>Train health workers |

*(Continued)*

*Table 6.1* (Continued)

| Authors | Country | Major Event | Main Pharmacists' Roles |
|---|---|---|---|
| Thompson CA.[52] | US | 2013 Oklahoma tornado | Temporary pharmacy set-up and services<br>Manage donated medicines |
| Ford H, Trent S, Wickizer S.[53] | US | 2015 Train derailed Blount County | Medication management<br>Information resource |
| Melin K, Maldonado WT, López-Candales A.[54] | Puerto Rico | 2017 Hurricane Maria | Medication management |
| Moss A, Green T, Moss S, et al.[55] | Australia | 2019/20 Bushfires | Medication management<br>Information resource<br>Triage<br>Prescribing<br>Coping with power outages<br>Managing people's emotions |

later in 1852.[1] However, the separation of pharmacy as a distinct profession independent from medicine had barely commenced when the war began in 1861. Interestingly, nursing as a profession was not yet established at all and the war is attributed to helping solidify it into its own viable profession in the United States.[1] Without large manufacturing warehouses or large pharmaceutical companies, unsurprisingly the main role of pharmacists in the 1800s was compounding and manufacturing of medicines. They focused on ensuring the quality of ingredients and accuracy of compounding and prescriptions. Additionally pharmacists worked as 'hospital stewards' who would dispense and compound the medicines prescribed by physicians.[1] The education pharmacists received was varied and it was largely considered to be a trade requiring on-the-job training as opposed to the more formal education as it is today.

### World War I and II

The next account is of pharmacists' roles and services in the US military during the World Wars. This was published in 1966 by Charles Braucher, a pharmacist who served in the US army during World War II.[2] He described that in World War I, pharmacist roles included performing auxiliary medical roles. During World War II, those close to the action recognised that there were shortages for personnel to fulfil many necessary medical roles and thus saw the potential of including pharmacists to backfill these valuable roles. Some pharmacists were trained as 'assistant battalion surgeon' that were stationed at the back of the fighting battalion and involved providing first aid and first response to those injured.[2] The US Navy took a similar approach and had their 'Pharmacist's Mate Standing Watch' prepared and trained as first responders to care for the injured and sick until other medical services were available.[2]

Interestingly, at the same time on their home soil in the United States, pharmacists were not quite valued in the same way. In 1944 after a fire in Cleveland, US pharmacists were identified as having treated and provided first aid to affected individuals before other medical services could arrive.[2] They were acknowledged and thanked by the Mayor of the region for their emergency service in a statement that reads,

> *these men by their quick thinking and action, their ability to respond with calmness and courage in the face of an emergency, and their application of professional skill with no thought of personal reward or recognition, deserve the thanks of communities everywhere.*[2]

However, the Chief Medical Officer at the time and the American Pharmaceutical Association disagreed with pharmacists assuming a first responder type role and consequently stated that the main role of pharmacists should remain logistics and medicine supply.[2] Sadly, after World

War II ended and there was no more pressure to meet a critical medical need, the advancement pharmacists had made in the US military as first responders was all but forgotten.

### Anthrax Crisis

A key role that is more specific to bioterrorism is prophylaxis management. No one does mass distribution of medications better than pharmacists. Unsurprisingly, people are scared when they are told that they have been exposed to something that is hazardous to their health and they have a lot of questions. People are complex and many have comorbidities or circumstances that may impact the type of medication they receive. Pharmacists are key to lead the development of treatment algorithms, counsel patients on the use of prophylactic medicines, and to answer questions (e.g., can I take this with my other medications? Can I take this if I'm pregnant or breastfeeding? Can my child take this medication?).

The 2001 anthrax crisis in Washington D.C. in the United States, saw pharmacists take a leadership role in the screening process to determine treatment or prophylaxis choice based on other patient determinants such as pregnancy status, other medical conditions, ongoing medications, and allergies.[56] The 2001 Anthrax scare has seen a role emerge for pharmacists in bioterrorism prevention and preparedness. It also highlighted the important role that pharmacists have as the reliable and trusted source of evidence-based information for specifics about the emergency event, impact on the community, response measures, and recovery steps. This has led to some pharmacy organisations suggesting pharmacists should become more involved in bioterrorism preparation, remaining up-to-date with the current threats and management solutions.[23,57]

A study by Brown, Doyle, and Ojo in 2008, assessed the knowledge and training of English pharmacists for CBRN disasters.[58] They identified that pharmacists knowledge and ability to recognise and manage CBRN disasters was low. However, over half of the participants believed that CBRN training should be included in undergraduate or postgraduate training for pharmacists. So, there was a high willingness of pharmacists to learn and be more involved in CBRN management.[58]

### Hurricane Katrina

Hurricane Katrina was extremely destructive when it that struck the Gulf states of the United States (Texas, Louisiana, Alabama, Mississippi, and Florida). It made landfall as a Category 4 (second highest category of the Saffir–Simpson storm scale) on August 29, 2005.[59] In the midst of this hurricane, the affected US state of Alabama temporarily extended its 'emergency supply' rule allowing pharmacists to prescribe a 30-day emergency supply of chronic condition medications for disaster-affected patients without a prescription. Alabama State also permitted the use of out-of-state volunteer pharmacists to assist in the relief efforts.[60,61] This is highlighted in the below quote,

> *... in the aftermath of the hurricane, it quickly became clear that pharmacist assistance and medications were critically needed in the areas affected by the storm as well as those states sheltering evacuees.*[28]

In its aftermath, pharmacists assisted in the healthcare clinics set up in evacuation centres to reduce the strain on local hospitals. Hospitals had been inundated with disaster-affected individuals not requiring immediate medical assistance.[37,59] Many evacuees required replacement medications as they left their homes with only enough for 1–2 days' supply, or in the case of evacuation to the Louisiana Superdome, patients with their medications packed in weekly pill boxes, had their medications confiscated and destroyed as part of the registration protocol.[59,62–64] Pharmacists performed many duties in the wake of Hurricane Katrina and fulfilled new roles in the absence of other healthcare professionals.[65] Some of the duties pharmacists performed following Hurricane Katrina included[37,65–68]

- triaging and first responder services within evacuation centres (separating those patients needing to see a doctor from those who simply needed a prescription refill, and identifying and referring individuals to allied health professionals),
- taking medication histories,
- providing vaccinations,
- performing basic medical checks,
- mixing intravenous medications,
- providing consultations on wound infections,
- assisting with major traumas,
- assessing the safety of medications brought in against contamination, and
- pill identification.

### Great East Japan Earthquake

The Great East Japan Earthquake that occurred in 2011 is an example of the cascading effect of natural hazards. It started with an earthquake that caused a tsunami and flash flood that set off a nuclear event.[69] This disaster highlighted the effects resulting from poor disaster management and the need to apply a systems thinking lens.[69,70] The inability of the organisations (i.e., government, power plant operator, disaster planners) involved to analyse all the potential outcomes of policy changes led to a natural hazard causing the cascading effect.[69]

Japanese pharmacists were integral in the emergency response to this disaster. Pharmacists and pharmacy students volunteer their services to sort through medicines and relief supplies and ensured they were being appropriately stored. They were also first responders with some being redeployed from their usual practice settings to contribute as clinical members of the DMATs.[47] It was also reported that pharmacy students were volunteering and backfilling pharmacist roles to free them up to undertake other roles. It was also highlighted that pharmacists need education on emergency management of nuclear disasters, as it was evident that they were unsure how to prescribe, manage, and counsel on potassium iodide.

It cannot be ignored that major emergencies like these have a significant personal toll and loss on those that are responding and yet, pharmacists that are placed in these incredibly difficult situations continue to help. Mr Tanno, a Japanese pharmacist, was personally affected by The Great East Japan Earthquake when his pharmacy was being completely destroyed.[49] But that and his personal trauma and loss didn't stop him from wading out in the waist-deep water and mud to offer his assistance. He set-up temporary pharmacy services in the school that was rapidly being transformed into an evacuation centre and offered his assistance in the nearby hospital. Mr Tanno put it simply, *"The pharmacists work for the people in the community, not for themselves. He wishes to see a return to that community way of thinking and hopes that future pharmacists will share in this vision"*.[49]

With the number of disasters experienced by Japanese pharmacists, emergency management has begun to be incorporated into one of their university's undergraduate pharmacy curriculum as an entirely separate division or speciality for the school of pharmacy.[71]

### SARS Pandemics

Pharmacists (community and hospital) were of great assistance during the Severe Acute Respiratory Syndrome (SARS) outbreak of 2003 which significantly affected parts of the world including Toronto in Ontario, Canada.[24,25] The local hospitals quickly put together multidisciplinary SARS teams that included pharmacists to treat the affected patients and limit the potential spread of the virus.[24] Pharmacists assisted in the screening of all presenting patients, provided medication expertise on best evidence-based treatment options to follow, and suggested dose adjustments to make.[24] Pharmacists with training in intensive care units (ICU) were training other pharmacists in a piggyback approach to increase the number of pharmacists available to assist in managing the ICU patients with SARS.

Due to the severity and contagious nature of the SARS virus, some hospitals and clinics were forced into quarantine, leaving patients with no tertiary healthcare service to turn to, relying on their local community pharmacies.[25] This placed considerable stress on both patients and pharmacists, as patients were unable to comprehend how, with no other alternative medical service available, the pharmacist was unable to assist in diagnosing and prescribing due to legal constraints and pharmacists were at a loss as to how to best assist their patients legally.[25]

Looking at the impact on community pharmacists, Austin and colleagues completed a study where they interviewed pharmacists that worked on the frontline during SARS. The community pharmacists expressed concerns regarding working without documented policies and procedures in place as they did not feel equipped to handle the challenging working conditions brought on by the SARS outbreak and a power outage.[25] Older, more experienced pharmacists were more willing to assist their patients in the absence of documented policies and procedures. They recalled the days of handwriting labels and manually checking drug interactions before the advent of computer software. They were able to think on their feet in order to service their communities during the crisis.[25] Austin and colleagues identified that newer graduates preferred to follow protocols and procedures strictly to the letter in their day-to-day practice. They were less willing to rely on their own professional judgement and therefore struggled to adapt their practice to the changed working conditions brought about by the disasters.[25]

### Fort McMurray Wildfires

During the Calgary floods and Fort McMurray wildfires, pharmacists were increasingly being sought after for their clinical expertise.[72] In the case of Fort McMurray, the Alberta Health Services' pharmacy leadership made the suggestion to their upper management for the utilisation of pharmacist assessing and prescribing services.[72] Pharmacists were integral to assessing and prescribing for patients in the evacuation centres. They were also required to join the field hospital set up by the military and asked to assess and triage patients. It was not only the displaced and disaster-affected individuals that pharmacists helped but also the volunteer firefighters who suffered from smoke inhalation or ran out of their medications.[72]

### Thunderstorm Asthma

Pharmacists also provided vital assistance during the thunderstorm asthma event which occurred on November 21st and 22nd in Melbourne, Australia in 2016. Thunderstorm asthma is a particular type of asthma triggered by an uncommon combination of high pollen (usually during late Spring to early Summer) and a specific type of thunderstorm.[73] With this storm event, grass pollen grains are swept up into clouds as the storm forms. These pollen grains subsequently absorb moisture causing them to burst open releasing large amounts of smaller allergen particles. One pollen grain can potentially release up to 700 of these smaller allergenic particles which are sufficiently small enough to penetrate human airways. People who suffer from allergic rhinitis (hay fever) and/or asthma are particularly susceptible to respiratory problems during these events.[73]

During this event, health services were inundated with people experiencing respiratory problems and unfortunately nine people lost their lives.[74] Hospital EDs were overcrowded with 9,909 people who presented to public hospitals, 231 presented to private hospitals, and many others who self-presented to community pharmacies.[74] There were 2,666 calls made to paramedics and ambulance services, of which 962 related to respiratory problems.[74] This thunderstorm asthma epidemic was referred to in the media as having an equivalent impact to a terrorist attack.[75] The Victorian state government issued a review into the thunderstorm asthma event and subsequent healthcare response, which was conducted by the Inspector-General for Emergency Management (IGEM) for the state of Victoria. The IGEM review produced recommendations on ways the health systems could be better prepared to respond to an unknown event like the thunderstorm asthma epidemic.[74] Recommendation three from the IGEM review suggests public health systems need to learn to

> … *work with primacy care providers including appropriate community pharmacy representatives to consider and define the role community pharmacies play during emergencies and where appropriate, integrate community pharmacies into future planning for emergencies.*[74] *(p.5)*

The IGEM report suggests that health systems need to broaden their governance arrangements to include pharmacists and pharmacies.[74] This report highlights the significant role pharmacists and pharmacies played in providing care to patients during this event. There were large numbers of people presenting to community pharmacies due to the wait times in the EDs at the hospitals.[74] Finding Six from the IGEM report states:

> *IGEM finds that on 21–22 November 2016 community pharmacies played a central role in meeting community needs during the thunderstorm asthma event. Given their community focus and their geographic coverage, community pharmacies can provide valuable support to the management of health emergencies or emergencies with health impacts.*[74] *(p.36)*

In sharing the responsibility for preparing and mitigating the health impacts of a disaster, the IGEM report proposes pharmacists and pharmacies belong as part of the health sector main stakeholder group.[74]

## Australian 2019–2020 Bushfires

The Australian Black Sumer bushfires that occurred in the summer of 2019-2020 were extensive in impact and reach. It impacted almost every state and territory in Australia and burnt over 17 million hectares of land.[76,77] While not the deadliest Australian bushfire, it became the worst bushfire season on record for New South Wales (NSW) with 6.7% of the state being burnt including 37% of the state's national park land.[76,77]

A study of this event reported the inflexibility of legislation preventing pharmacists from operating outside of the pharmacy building (even after appealing for an exemption).[55] So, every morning the pharmacists went to the evacuation centre and found out from the attending medical staff what was needed, drove back to the pharmacy to dispense the necessary medications, and collect the required items (e.g., baby formula, bottles, reading glasses, over-the-counter medications, walking aids, diapers, etc.), then drove back to the evacuation centre at lunchtime to deliver them to the patients. Then they would repeat this ritual in the afternoon. I've heard countless stories from pharmacists of similar frustrations and feeling hindered to fulfil their roles by pharmacy legislation.

## Evolution of Pharmacists' Roles in Disasters

We have covered a lot of events and pharmacists' roles that have changed over the past several decades. So, let's put it together. Figure 6.1 is an

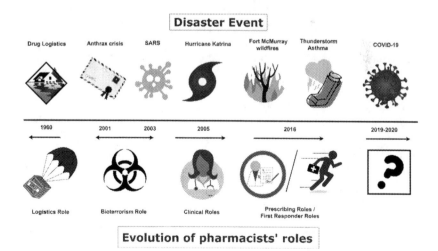

*Figure 6.1* Evolution of pharmacists' roles in disasters and emergencies. Originally published in *Canadian Pharmacists Journal* and reproduced with permission.[72]

illustration of the evolution of pharmacists' roles in disasters and emergencies across some big events in specific regions.[72,78] With each passing event, there is a trend of greater recognition of pharmacists' unique contributions to disaster health management.

Prior to the events of 9/11 in the United States, pharmacists' roles in relation to disasters were strongly linked to their expertise in logistics and getting medicines from A to B.[78] After the events of 9/11 in 2001 in the United States and the SARS epidemic in 2003, pharmacists were acknowledged for their drug expertise and contributions in bioterrorism emergencies and pandemics. In 2005, Hurricane Katrina significantly impacted regions of the United States and highlighted the valuable pharmacists' roles in providing clinical services to disaster-affected communities. In 2016, two specific events in different parts of the world—Canada and Australia—ignited the recognition of pharmacists' essential role in being a first responder in disasters and emergencies providing clinical pharmacy services (e.g., prescribing, assessing, triaging, etc.).[78]

This figure was designed at the very beginning of the COVID-19 pandemic in 2020 and thus, we did not know what kind of impact it would have and how it would contribute to our timeline. Now, more than two years into the pandemic, we are getting a better sense of pharmacists' roles and the impact the COVID-19 pandemic is having on the pharmacy profession.

## The COVID-19 Pandemic

Pharmacists have once again stepped up to meet the needs. They have continued to provide the steady, reliable, and accessible evidence-based healthcare to the community during the COVID-19 pandemic that we have come to expect. My team conducted a survey on the impact of the COVID-19 pandemic on Canadian frontline pharmacists.[79] This study identified frontline pharmacists' roles being performed and the challenges being faced during the early phase of the pandemic (March–July 31, 2020). Out of 740 Canadian pharmacists that responded, 72% stated they had patients and members of the public coming to pharmacies for care while avoiding other healthcare avenues out of fear of contracting the COVID-19 infection.[79] The increased pressure this placed on pharmacists was not only from patients seeking medications or health services, but 59% of the pharmacists surveyed stated they had members of the public seeking information about the COVID-19 pandemic and public health measures.[79] Furthermore, 53% of them also stated members of the public were coming to the pharmacy to have a pharmacist calm their fears and anxiety about COVID-19.[79] These statistics highlight the remarkable trust and respect community members place in their pharmacists for their unbiased and evidence-based knowledge and their reliance on pharmacy services during emergencies.

It is important to recognise that pharmacies were unable to close and readjust like other healthcare entities, they had to remain open and figure out their emergency response based upon the limited information that was available in the early days of the pandemic. The major challenges these pharmacists initially faced was accessing personal protective equipment (PPE) supplies,[79] as they were not initially included in the government procurement allotment and yet they were on the frontline where all types of patients mix – the healthy, the sick, and the at-risk. Another challenge these pharmacists faced in the early days of the pandemic, was rationing of medications in order to combat the medication shortages and ensure ongoing and equitable access.[79]

Prior to the COVID-19 pandemic, the majority (76%) of Canadian pharmacists surveyed were not engaged in local disaster and emergency management response or planning.[79] This signifies a serious disconnect between the essential frontline disaster roles being performed by our pharmacists and pharmacies within our communities' emergency response planning. This raises the question, on the heels of our collective pandemic experiences, are we as the global pharmacy profession capitalising on this to better engage our pharmacists in emergency management?

A recent scoping review conducted by our team highlighted the vast array of pharmacists' roles and services provided worldwide during the first year of the COVID-19 pandemic.[78] There were 63 articles published in 2020 that made 570 references to the roles and services of frontline pharmacists. Interestingly, the most discussed role was interprofessional collaboration.[78] As pharmacists, we are our patient's advocate, working in tandem with other professions to achieve the patient's goals. Another highly discussed role was education[78] and this is a core skill of pharmacists as we are not only experts in evaluating evidence (like evaluating the studies that were published about COVID treatments), but we are skilled in tailoring our communication to their different audiences – we can speak medical to our healthcare colleagues, policy to governments, and understandable and related language to our patients and community members. These roles and services that were visible during the pandemic were grouped into three main categories—public health, information, and medication management (Figure 6.2).[78] What was fascinating was the disparity of acknowledgement and acceptance of pharmacists' role across these three categories. Pharmacists' roles in medication management, which involves the smallest audience, and yet, it's the most widely recognised role attributed to pharmacists. At the other end of the scale are pharmacists' roles in public health, which are more visible at the global-health level and have the largest audience of society, yet are the least acknowledged or accepted pharmacists' roles and services.[78] We believe that COVID-19 has changed this with the enormous global scale and

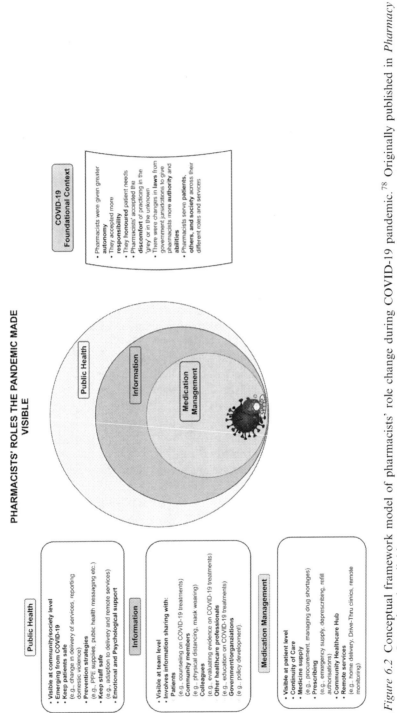
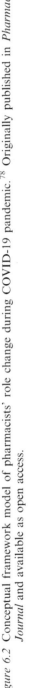

**PHARMACISTS' ROLES THE PANDEMIC MADE VISIBLE**

**COVID-19 Foundational Context**

- Pharmacists were given greater **autonomy**
- They accepted more **responsibility**
- They **honoured** patient needs
- Pharmacists' accepted the **discomfort** of practising in the 'grey' or in the unknown
- There were changes in **laws** from government jurisdictions to give pharmacists more **authority and abilities**
- Pharmacists serve **patients, others, and society** across their different roles and services

**Public Health**

- **Visible at community/society level**
- **Emerging from COVID-19**
- **Keep patients safe**
  (e.g., change in delivery of services, reporting domestic violence)
- **Prevention strategies**
  (e.g., PPE supplies, public health messaging etc.)
- **Keep staff safe**
  (e.g., adaption to delivery and remote services)
- **Emotional and Psychological support**

**Information**

- **Visible at team level**
- **Involves information sharing with:**
  **Patients**
  (e.g., counselling on COVID-19 treatments)
  **Community members**
  (e.g., physical distancing, mask wearing)
  **Colleagues**
  (e.g., evaluating evidence on COVID-19 treatments)
  **Other healthcare professionals**
  (e.g., education on COVID-19 treatments)
  **Government/organizations**
  (e.g., policy development)

**Medication Management**

- **Visible at patient level**
- **Continuity of Care**
- **Medicine supply**
  (e.g., procurement, managing drug shortages)
- **Prescribing**
  (e.g., emergency supply, deprescribing, refill authorisations)
- **Community Healthcare Hub**
- **Remote services**
  (e.g., home delivery, Drive-Thru clinics, remote monitoring)

*Figure 6.2* Conceptual framework model of pharmacists' role change during COVID-19 pandemic.[78] Originally published in *Pharmacy Journal* and available as open access.

prolonged nature of this crisis. It has made visible the changes to pharmacists' roles and services.

During COVID-19, pharmacists took this role to a new level with finding innovative ways to share this information with everyone by broadcasting on the radio and on television.[78] Pharmacists also provided numerous public health roles in asymptomatic COVID screening and testing, COVID vaccinations, managing access to PPE supplies, combatting misinformation about COVID transmission, and treatments.[78] Other more established roles that pharmacists provide were publicised as pharmacists compounded hand sanitizer and managed drug shortages.

What I find truly fascinating about the COVID-19 pandemic, is the widespread acceptance and recognition of the amazing roles and services pharmacists have been providing. Pharmacists are finally receiving the long-held desire of their middle child that craved confirmation of their role in public health and emergencies. And this could lead to a new era of pharmacy. But more on this in Chapter 19.

## Chapter References

1 Flannery MA Civil War pharmacy: a history of drugs, drug supply and provision, and therapeutics for the Union and Confederacy. New York: Pharmaceutical Products Press; 2004.

2 Braucher CL The mission of the pharmacist in nuclear disaster. *Mil. Med.* 1966; 131(3):234–244.

3 MacCara ME Combatting Spanish influenza: Focus on pharmacists, pharmacies and drugs. *Canadian Pharmacists Journal/Revue des Pharmaciens du Canada* 2020; 153(6):335–342.

4 Scott S, Constantine LM When Natural Disaster Strikes: With careful planning, pharmacists can continue to provide essential services to survivors in the aftermath of a disaster. *Am. Pharm.* 1990; 30(11):27–31.

5 Grabenstein JD Public and patient concerns in catastrophic circumstances. *Am. J. Health Syst. Pharm.* 2002; 59(10):923–925.

6 Cramer R, Weeks K Pharmacy disaster emergency: the Huntsville tornado. *Hosp. Pharm.* 1990; 25(6):523–526.

7 Carda E, Harcum J, Olthoff C Mass casualty: a hospital pharmacist's call to action. *Hosp. Pharm.* 1989; 24(9):697–698, 712.

8 Nestor A, Aviles AI, Kummerle DR, Barclay LP, Rey JA Pharmaceutical services at a medical site after Hurricane Andrew. *Am. J. Hosp. Pharm.* 1993; 50(9):1896–1898.

9 Merges V Hurricane Iniki--providing hospital pharmacy services. *Hosp. Pharm.* 1993; 28(5):393–394, 400.

10 Miller C Hurricane Iniki--providing Prescription Service in a Clinic. *Hosp. Pharm.* 1993; 28(5):401–403.

11 Bussières J-F, St-Arnaud C, Schunck C, Lamarre D, Jouberton F The role of the pharmacist in humanitarian aid in Bosnia-Herzegovina: the experience of Pharmaciens Sans Frontieres. *Ann. Pharmacother.* 2000; 34(1):112–118.

12 Lambert E Humanitarian aid in Casamance. *Pharm. J.* 2008; 281(7533):756.

13 Bethea S Pharmacy mass casualty disaster plan implemented after the train wreck. *Hosp. Pharm.* 1994; 29(3):224–225.

14 Leduc D, Levy D DMAT pharmacies. *Emergency* 1994; 26:18–23.

15 Sagraves R Pharmacists are heroes, too. *Am. Pharm.* 1995; NS35(10):33–34.

16 Burda AM, Sigg T Pharmacy preparedness for incidents involving weapons of mass destruction. *Am. J. Health Syst. Pharm.* 2001; 58(23):2274–2284.

17 Berod T, Chan-ou-Teung F Pharmacist's role in rescue efforts after plane crash in Indian Ocean. *Am. J. Health Syst. Pharm.* 1997; 54(9):1110–.

18 Montello MJ, Ostroff C, Frank EC, Haffer AS, James RR 2001 Anthrax crisis in Washington, DC: Pharmacists' role in screening patients and selecting prophylaxis. *Am. J. Health Syst. Pharm.* 2002; 59(12):1193–1199.

19 Haffer AS, James RR, Montello MJ, Frank EC, Ostroff C 2001 Anthrax crisis in Washington, DC: Clinic for persons exposed to contaminated mail. *Am. J. Health Syst. Pharm.* 2002; 59(12):1189–1192.

20 Babb J, Downs K Fighting back: pharmacists' roles in the federal response to the September 11 attacks. *J. Am. Pharm. Assoc. (Wash.)* 2001; 41(6):834–837.

21 Gaudette R, Schnitzer J, George E, Briggs SM Lessons learned from the September 11th World Trade Center disaster: pharmacy preparedness and participation in an international medical and surgical response team. *Pharmacotherapy: The Journal of Human Pharmacology and Drug Therapy* 2002; 22(3):271–281.

22 Babb J, Tosatto R, Hayslett J Disaster planning and emergency preparedness: lessons learned. *Journal of the American Pharmaceutical Association* (Washington, DC: 1996) 2002; 42(5 Suppl 1):S50–S51.

23 Cohen V Organization of a Health-System Pharmacy Team to Respond to Episodes of Terrorism. *Am. J. Health Syst. Pharm.* 2003; 60(12):1257.

24 Chin TWF, Chant C, Tanzini R, Wells J Severe Acute Respiratory Syndrome (SARS): The Pharmacist's Role. *Pharmacotherapy* 2004; 24(6):705–712.

25 Austin Z, Martin JC, Gregory PA Pharmacy Practice in Times of Civil Crisis: The Experience of SARs and "The Blackout" in Ontario, Canada. *Research in Social and Administrative Pharmacy* 2007; 3(3):320–335.

26 Mason P Tsunami relief: same mistakes repeated. *Pharm. J.* 2005; 274(7336): 178–.

27 Kirtley JC Pharmacy's dedication in meeting hurricane evacuees' needs. *J. Am. Pharm. Assoc.* (2003) 2005; 45(6):653.

28 Lynas K Pharmacists answer the call in wake of Hurricane Katrina. *Canadian Pharmacists Journal* 2005; 138(7):17.

29 Velazquez L, Dallas S, Rose L, Evans KS, Saville R, Wang J, et al. A PHS pharmacist team's response to Hurricane Katrina. *Am. J. Health Syst. Pharm.* 2006; 63(14):1332–1335.

30 Russum M Responding to Katrina: A Veterans Affairs pharmacist's experience. *Am. J. Health Syst. Pharm.* 2006; 63(9):809–810.

31 Henderson GS Finding Supplies. *N. Engl. J. Med.* 2005; 353(15):1542–.

32 Geraci SA, Douglas S, Algood TL, Pinkston W, Sanders S, Kirchner K Hurricane Katrina: the Jackson veterans Affairs Medical Center experience. *The American journal of the medical sciences* 2008; 336(2):116–123.

33 Kaldy J Hurricane Katrina: pharmacists reflect on lessons learned. *The Consultant Pharmacist®* 2007; 22(3):199–211.

34 Young D Pharmacists play vital roles in Katrina response: more disaster-response participation urged. Oxford University Press; 2005.
35 Bratberg J Hurricane Katrina: pharmacists making a difference: a Rhode Island pharmacist shares his Gulf Coast experiences as part of a disaster-relief team. *J. Am. Pharm. Assoc.* (2003) 2005; 45(6):654–658.
36 Bethea S Reflections from a Director of Pharmacy Dealing with Hurricane Katrina. Los Angeles, CA: SAGE Publications Sage CA; 2005.
37 Hogue MD, Hogue HB, Lander RD, Avent K, Fleenor M The Non Traditional Role of Pharmacists After Hurricane Katrina: Process Description and Lessons Learned. *Public Health Rep.* 2009; 124(2):217–223.
38 Jhung MA, Shehab N, Rohr-Allegrini C, Pollock DA, Sanchez R, Guerra F, et al. Chronic Disease and Disasters. Medication Demands of Hurricane Katrina Evacuees. *Am. J. Prev. Med.* 2007; 33(3):207–210.
39 Lust E Caring for Animal Patients Following Hurricane Katrina: People weren't the only ones stranded and traumatized by events on the Gulf Coast. *J. Am. Pharm. Assoc.* (2003) 2005; 45(6):659–662.
40 Labdi BA Working with hurricane Rita. *Am. J. Health Syst. Pharm.* 2006; 63(21):2053–2054.
41 Gershgol SM, Cantrell L, Mutrux B Disaster relief efforts of pharmacy students during California wildfires. *Am. J. Health Syst. Pharm.* 2008; 65(21): 2006–2007.
42 Bhavsar TR, Kim H-J, Yu Y Roles and contributions of pharmacists in regulatory affairs at the Centers for Disease Control and Prevention for public health emergency preparedness and response. *J. Am. Pharm. Assoc.* (2003) 2010; 50(2):165–168.
43 Schwerzmann J, Graitcer SB, Jester B, Krahl D, Jernigan D, Bridges CB, et al. Evaluating the impact of pharmacies on pandemic influenza vaccine administration. *Disaster Med. Public Health Prep.* 2017; 11(5):587–593.
44 Huynh C, Lott A Lessons from a service learning trip to Haiti. *Am. J. Health Syst. Pharm.* 2011; 68(3):196–200.
45 Ferris D Pharmacist's assistance after Haiti earthquake. *Am. J. Health Syst. Pharm.* 2010; 67(14):1138–1141.
46 Hashimoto T, Sato H Earthquake, tsunami, and pharmaceutical care in eastern Japan. *J. Am. Pharm. Assoc.* (2003) 2011; 51(5):568.
47 Takeda Y A report from Japan: disaster relief efforts of pharmacists in response to the Great East Japan Earthquake. *SA Pharmaceutical Journal* 2011; 78(9):42–46.
48 Kawataba Y Considerations for pharmacists working in major disaster areas. *International journal of pharmaceutical compounding* 2013; 17(6):459–463.
49 Epp DA, Tanno Y, Brown A, Brown B Pharmacists' reactions to natural disasters:From Japan to Canada. *Can Pharm J (Ott)* 2016; 149(4):204–215.
50 Mak PW, Singleton J Burning Questions: Exploring the Impact of Natural Disasters on Community Pharmacies. *Research in Social and Administrative Pharmacy* 2017; 13(1):162–171.
51 Erickson K An emergency department pharmacist's experience at the Boston Marathon. *Am. J. Health Syst. Pharm.* 2013; 70(19):1652–1654.
52 Thompson CA Oklahoma community recovers through pharmacists' help. Oxford University Press; 2013.

53  Ford H, Trent S, Wickizer S Pharmacy Services After a Tank Car Derailment and Toxic Chemical Release in Blount County, Tennessee. *J. Am. Pharm. Assoc.* (2003) 2017; 57(1):56–61.e2.

54  Melin K, Maldonado WT, López-Candales A Lessons learned from Hurricane Maria: pharmacists' perspective. *Ann. Pharmacother.* 2018; 52(5):493–494.

55  Moss A, Green T, Moss S, Waghorn J, Bushell MJ Exploring Pharmacists' Roles during the 2019-2020 Australian Black Summer Bushfires. *Pharmacy (Basel)* 2021; 9(3).

56  Haffer A, Rogers J, Montello MJ, Frank EC, Ostroff C 2001 Anthrax Crisis in Washington, DC: Pharmacists' Role in Screening Patients and Selecting Prophylaxis. *Am. J. Health Syst. Pharm.* 2002; 59(12):1193–1199.

57  American Society of Health-System Pharmacists (ASHP). ASHP Statement on the Role of Health-System Pharmacists in Emergency Preparedness. *Am. J. Health Syst. Pharm.* 2003; 60(19):1993.

58  Brown D, Doyle P, Ojo R An assessment of the training, knowledge and understanding of terrorism countermeasures among British pharmacists. *Pharm. J.* 2008; 281:133–137.

59  Currier M, King DS, Wofford MR, Daniel BJ A Katrina Experience: Lessons Learned. *Am. J. Med.* 2006; 119(11):986–992.

60  Traynor K Pharmacy, Public Health Intersect in Alabama Disaster Plans. *Am. J. Health Syst. Pharm.* 2007; 64(19):1998–1999.

61  Ford JH Pharmacists in Disasters [PhD Thesis]. Athens, Gerogia: University of Georgia; 2013.

62  Kleinpeter MA, Norman LD, Krane NK Dialysis Services in the Hurricane-Affected Areas in 2005: Lessons Learned. *Am. J. Med. Sci.* 2006; 332(5): 259–263.

63  Miller AC, Arquilla B Chronic Diseases and Natural Hazards: Impact of Disasters on Diabetic, Renal, and Cardiac Patients. *Prehosp. Disaster Med.* 2008; 23(02):185–194.

64  Carameli KA, Eisenman DP, Blevins J, d'Angona B, Glik DC Planning for Chronic Disease Medications in Disaster: Perspectives from Patients, Physicians, Pharmacists, and Insurers. *Disaster Med. Public Health Prep.* 2013; 7(3):257–265.

65  Young D Pharmacists Play Vital Roles in Katrina Response More Disaster-Response Participation Urged. *Am. J. Health Syst. Pharm.* 2005; 62(21): 2202–2216.

66  Velazquez L, Dallas S, Rose L, Eva KS, Saville R, Wang J, et al. A PHS Pharmacist Team's Response to Hurricane Katrina. *Am. J. Health Syst. Pharm.* 2006; 63(14).

67  Angelo LB, Maffeo CM. Local and Global Volunteer Opportunities for Pharmacists to Contribute to Public Health. *Int. J. Pharm. Pract.* 2011; 19(3):206–213.

68  Pedersen CA, Canaday BR, Ellis WM, Keyes EK, Pietrantoni A, Rothholz MC, et al. Pharmacists' Opinions Regarding Level of Involvement in Emergency Preparedness and Response. *J. Am. Pharm. Assoc.* (2003) 2003; 43(6):694–701.

69  Cavallo A, Ireland V Preparing for Complex Interdependent Risks: A System of Systems Approach to Building Disaster Resilience. *International journal of disaster risk reduction* 2014; 9:181–193.

70 Takeda Y A Report from Japan: Disaster Relief Efforts of Pharmacists in Response to the Great East Japan Earthquake. *SA Pharmaceutical Journal (sapj)* 2011; 78(9):42–46.

71 Moriyama Y OKADAI Model as Disaster Medicine Education in Pharmacy Education: Mission and Road Map of the School of Pharmacy. *Yakugaku zasshi: Journal of the Pharmaceutical Society of Japan* 2014; 134(1):17–18.

72 Watson KE, Van Haaften D, Horon K, Tsuyuki RT The evolution of pharmacists' roles in disasters, from logistics to assessing and prescribing. *Can Pharm J (Ott)* 2020; 153(3):129–131.

73 Asthma Australia. Thunderstorm Asthma [Internet]. Victoria: Department of Health and Human Services, Asthma Australia, Australasian Society of Clinical Immunology and Allergy (ASCIA),; 2017 [cited 2018 18th Nov]; Available from: http://www.webcitation.org/76JsZ8lvC

74 Inspector-General for Emergency Management (IGEM), Victorian Government. Review of Response to the Thunderstorm Asthma Event of 21–22 November 2016: Final Report. 2017.

75 Davey M Thunderstorm Asthma: 'You're Talking an Event Equivalent to a Terrorist Attack' [Internet]. The Guardian Australian Edition; 2016 [cited 2018 28th Oct]; Available from: http://www.webcitation.org/73V3R3igi

76 Australian Institute for Disaster Resilience (AIDR). Major Incidents Report 2019–20 Department of Home Affairs. AIDR; 2020.

77 Richards L, Brew N, Smith L 2019–20 Australian bushfires—frequently asked questions: a quick guide [Internet]. Parliament of Australia,; 2020 [cited 2022 July 6]; Available from: https://www.aph.gov.au/About_Parliament/Parliamentary_Departments/Parliamentary_Library/pubs/rp/rp1920/Quick_Guides/AustralianBushfires

78 Watson KE, Schindel TJ, Barsoum ME, Kung JY COVID the Catalyst for Evolving Professional Role Identity? A Scoping Review of Global Pharmacists' Roles and Services as a Response to the COVID-19 Pandemic. *Pharmacy* 2021; 9(2):99.

79 Lee DH, Watson KE, Al Hamarneh YN Impact of COVID-19 on frontline pharmacists' roles and services in Canada: The INSPIRE Survey. *Can Pharm J (Ott)* 2021; 0(0):17151635211028253.

# 7 PPRR Cycle and Pharmacists' Roles

## Introduction

In Chapter 5 we introduced the Disaster Pharmacy Model and discussed how pharmacists' roles span the four broad categories of – logistics, public health, patient care, and governance. In this chapter, we are going to break this down and look at the specific roles across the PPRR (prevention, preparedness, response, and recovery) emergency management cycle as agreed by a consensus panel of international experts in emergency management and healthcare.

It is important to identify and discuss the PPRR cycle as our roles do not begin after an emergency has impacted our community. In actual fact, our roles in emergency management never stop. We should always be working on disaster risk reduction strategies and preparing our communities to increase our collective resilience. The roles and services we provide during our response to a disaster, should be implemented and included in the collaborative disaster health plan and strategy. Without proper preparedness, the response will be inappropriate. As stated by an experienced disaster pharmacist, Pharmacists fit across the entire cycle,

> ... because we're not just talking natural disasters, we're talking about emerging infectious disease, potential violent terrorism, potential chemical weapons, all of those kinds of things as well. Pharmacists have an essential role. [115][1]

## PPRR Cycle

The health needs of disaster-affected society change over the course of a disaster. Therefore, our roles as pharmacists and pharmacy personnel need to adapt to meet these changing needs. Emergency management and disaster health management are typically discussed in terms of the PPRR cycle consisting of the four distinct phases – prevention/mitigation/readiness, preparedness, response, and recovery.[2,3]

DOI: 10.4324/b23292-9

The term phases can imply there is a linear relationship between the phases in the cycle and that they occur consecutively. However, in actuality each phase is interlinked and occurs simultaneously – adapting and moulding to meet the requirements presented by the unique disaster or emegency.[4] When a linear relationship is assumed, the overlapping or simultaneous nature of the PPRR 'phases' can be lost in our interpretation and we may not action our response or recovery plans in a timely manner.

Figure 7.1 illustrates the two common ways in which the PPRR cycle is often discussed and illustrated. Currently, both models are required to fully comprehend the cyclic, overlapping, and simultaneous nature of the emergency management and disaster health management cycle.

I suggest a slightly different way of viewing the PPRR cycle, where these two images are essentially combined (Figure 7.2). It's important to understand that prevention/mitigation and preparedness are long-term processes. These phases do not stop once a disaster strikes but their respective tasks and duties continue throughout a disaster event. Comparably, the response phase is not just a reaction to the emergency but requires pre-empting the event (where possible) and putting into motion the disaster plans previously developed to ensure the response is effective. Similarly, recovery does not simply start after the conclusion of the response phase. These phases are overlapping and occur simultaneously, to give the most appropriate, cohesive, comprehensive, and coordinated disaster management strategy (Figure 7.2).

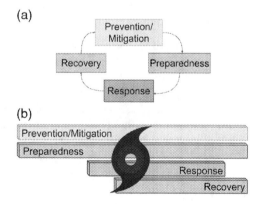

*Figure 7.1* (a) PPRR as four individual phases which occur as a continuous cycle, and (b) the PPRR cycle as a linear but overlapping process, where the phases are interlinked and occur simultaneously. The tornado icon signifies a disaster and each of the phases is illustrated as being when they would occur in relation to the disaster event.

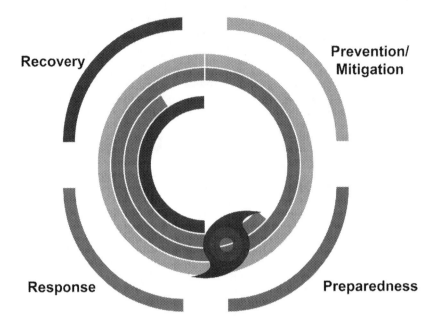

*Figure 7.2* PPRR illustrated as cyclic, overlapping, and simultaneous in nature. Prevention/mitigation (green) and preparedness (purple) phases are a continuous process, whereas response (orange) and recovery (blue) are engaged when a disaster occurs. The hurricane symbol represents the disaster event with time running clockwise.

## Prevention/Mitigation Phase

It can often be confusing to understand the prevention and mitigation stage, as surely, we cannot prevent a disaster or emergency from occurring. And, of course, you would be correct. However, what we can do is mitigate the impact a natural hazard has on our communities, reducing the risk of the hazard becoming a disaster in the first place and reducing the impact it has on people's health. These strategies also reduce the costs of our collective response and recovery efforts.[5] Prevention in terms of healthcare is seen as mitigating the health impacts of a disaster.[6,7] I really like the way Chan and colleagues state it, the purpose of prevention is,

> *To avoid increasing the burden of clinical consults in disaster after-math, the health needs of people with underlying chronic conditions (drugs, special diets) should be attended to avoid medical complications of their underlying conditions due to lack of management.*[6 (p.18)]

## Pharmacists' Roles in the Prevention/Mitigation Phase

So, for each of these phases I have outlined the roles that were agreed upon by the consensus panel and listed the ones that pertain most specifically to the prevention and mitigation phase of the emergency management cycle. These roles include:[8]

- *Administer vaccinations* – Protecting community members against diseases to prevent a potential pandemic (e.g., influenza or measles).
- *Educate the public* – Pharmacists have a responsibility to educate their patients and community members on public health measures to reduce the spread of infections.
- *Tailor 'point of care' messaging and inform patients of their risk* – Our patients with chronic conditions are at increased risk of experiencing exacerbations and complications during disasters. So, we have a duty to explain to them their increased individual risk and help them to prepare and plan for disasters.
- *Optimise medication supplies* – Ensuring adequate supplies for your pharmacy, pharmacy department, or organisation to be self-sufficient for the first 24–96 hours after a disaster. Also, we need to ensure patients have their own reserve of medications to see them through the initial phase of a disaster when community health services may be inaccessible.

## Preparedness Phase

Next is the preparedness phase and this involves improving the adaptive capacity and increases the resiliency of organisations and the community.[3,9] It also includes all the necessary tasks to get the workforce ready (e.g., training, team relationships, volunteers, roles, etc.).[10] This is where all our time and effort should be spent, so our response is appropriate and seamless. To put it another way, an Olympics team puts all their concerted efforts into the four years of preparation and training so they can perform at the best during the Olympics games. No team rocks up to the game having put no thought in or not carefully training prior to the event.

One of the ways as pharmacists we can help build the resilient capacity of our community, is through providing awareness and education regarding hazards prone to the area. Are people aware they live in a city near a fault line or in a common path of tornadoes? This is also the time for us to build the relationships with other sectors of the disaster health system, so they are aware of what pharmacy's plan is for responding and to share knowledge and experiences to strengthen our collective response. These relationships will be heavily relied upon during the response and recovery phases.

## Pharmacists' Roles in the Preparedness Phase

And I have outlined the roles that were agreed upon by the consensus panel that pertain most specifically to the preparedness phase of the emergency management cycle. There is some overlap with the prevention phase, but here we are focusing on prepping our communities, working on relationships, and training our teams. These roles include:[8]

- *Advocate and represent* – Pharmacists need to have a voice and be active participants on local, state, and national disaster committees and disaster health teams. Otherwise, we risk the response being inappropriate and not meeting the needs of our community.
- *Disaster and emergency plans* – An important part of our business continuity plans should include disaster health management. How will you continue operations and meeting the needs of the community? What are your expectations of yourself or your staff during a disaster?
- *Develop drug algorithms and treatment guidelines* – Pharmacists are in the best position to identify and develop guidelines or algorithms for the treatment and prophylaxis to diseases based on co-morbidities (e.g., antibiotics for anthrax exposure).
- *Identify at-risk patients* – Based on our regular dealings with our patients, we are in a prime location to identify and check-in on our at-risk individuals when a disaster occurs.
- *Protect uninterrupted supply* – Where feasible it is our responsibility to ensure we build relationships with our suppliers and the local disaster groups to identify other avenues for medication supplies in case of disaster impacting the main supply routes. This includes securing cold chain lines. What are the plans in case of power outage for refrigerated medicines?
- *Know how to access the National Pharmaceutical Stockpiles (NPS)* – Depending on your practice setting, you may not be directly involved in your jurisdiction government's dissemination of the NPS. But it is good for pharmacists to know what medications are typically keep as part of the NPS and who to contact if required. The NPS is also known as the Strategic National Stockpile or the National Emergency Strategic Stockpile.

## Response Phase

As we mentioned earlier, the response phase does not begin after a disaster event has occurred but should anticipate the event and appropriately respond (where possible).[3] We typically do not wait for the house to be completely on fire, before we start to take steps to put out the fire that started in the kitchen. The response phase puts into actions the plans developed during the preparedness phase. To go back to our analogy, our response to put out the kitchen fire relies on whether we pre-emptively bought fire blankets or a fire extinguisher for the house to use in a situation like this. Otherwise, we are limited in what resources we have available or need to wait for external supports to help us out. The response phase tasks are designed to address the short-term issues and basic human rights of those adversely affected by a disaster or emergency.[6]

## Pharmacists' Roles in the Response Phase

I have outlined the roles that were agreed upon by the consensus panel and that pertain most specifically to the response phase of the emergency management cycle. Not all the pharmacists' roles listed would be applicable to every emergency situation, as it would depend on the practice setting, community needs, and availability of other health professions. However, it's important to know that you could be expected to undertake any one of these roles during an emergency response within your regional scope of practice. These roles are grouped into three broad categories/purposes and they include:[8]

- *Continuity of care* – We have a responsibility to ensure access to medications for our patients during a disaster. This includes coordinating logistics, rationing/limiting supplies, prescribing and supplying ongoing chronic disease medications, dispensing medications and general pharmacy health related items, counselling patients, making therapeutic substitutions, attending clinical ward rounds, and monitoring or assisting in the release and allocation of national stockpiles if required.
- *Triage and manage low-acuity patients* – Pharmacists can manage the 'walking wounded' and triage disaster-affected individuals to assess their medical needs. This would include: medication reconciliation; providing referrals to others for further assessment and care; providing first aid, wound care, and cardiopulmonary resuscitation (CPR); pill identification; medication safety; and prescribing and administering vaccinations.
- *Advocacy* – Pharmacists have an obligation to promote pharmacists' place in disasters. This includes acting as a media liaison, advocating for appropriateness of donated medicines, engaging the pharmacy student workforce, and monitoring at-risk individuals.

**Recovery Phase**

The recovery phase is considered the most complex of the four phases in emergency management and can often be misunderstood.[11] I really like the way Lonne and colleagues states the purpose of recovery, they said

> *Recovery begins with preparedness and continues until recovery transforms into ongoing community development.*[11] *(p.230)*

The impacts from a disaster can last from days to decades depending on the level of resilience a community has developed in the preparedness phase.[3,9] The recovery phase also involves supporting the physical, emotional, social, and psychological wellbeing of the individuals affected by the disaster.[9] Recovery doesn't really end but morphs into the ongoing preparedness for the next emergency.

**Pharmacists' Roles in the Recovery Phase**

I have outlined the roles that were agreed upon by the consensus panel and that pertain most specifically to the recovery phase of the emergency management cycle. These roles would include:[8]

- *Participate in after-action reports* – It is key that we learn and adapt our disaster plans in the recovery phase based on the lessons learnt from a current disaster experience. This includes documenting and publishing your experiences of working through a disaster event.
- *Check in on vulnerable and at-risk groups* – We need to check in on our vulnerable and at-risk patients. These groups usually recover slower than other parts of the community due to their reliance on the community health services.
- *Inform local disaster management groups* – It is important that we link back into the local disaster groups we worked with during the preparedness and response phases and report what challenges faced the pharmacy profession and how we can better integrate and support the collective response to a disaster.
- *Restore order* – We need to restore our medication stock levels and patient records.

This is not an exhaustive or static list as with each disaster and emergency, pharmacists are needing to undertake various different roles. But it provides a great starting place in defining what pharmacists' roles in disasters should be and how to integrate pharmacists into emergency management and health teams. The above-described roles were part of a definition process undertaken with an international consensus panel using an all-hazard approach.

Interestingly, two roles that I believe are important for pharmacists to consider in the response and recovery phases did not reach consensus by the panel and they were; (1) making dose adjustments to existing therapeutic regimens where clinically necessary and (2) providing behavioural and mental health support following a disaster to patients and staff. I believe, pharmacists are already doing these two roles as the needs arise during emergencies but have yet to receive the recognition and acknowledgement for their services. This has especially been true during the COVID-19 pandemic as pharmacists have reported providing both of these roles. Pehaps, this has changed as the consensus panel study was completed prior to the global COVID-19 pandemic.

## Chapter References

1 Watson KE. The roles of pharmacists in disaster health management in natural and anthropogenic disasters. [Thesis]. QUT ePrints: Queensland University of Technology; 2019 Available from: https://eprints.qut.edu.au/130757/

2 Resilient Community Organisations. Emergency management: Prevention, preparedness, response & recovery [Internet]. Australian Government Initative, National Climate Change Adaption Research Facility,; 2015 [cited 2018 3rd November]; Available from: http://www.webcitation.org/73diZIqnD

3 Baird M. The "phases" of emergency management, background paper. Prepared for the Intermodal Freight Transportation Institute (ITFI) University of Memphis. Nashville: Vanderbilt Center for Transportation Research (VECTOR); 2010.

4 King D. Organisations in disaster. *Nat. Haz.* 2007; 40(3):657–665.

5 FitzGerald G. Chapter 12: Prevention and mitigation. In: FitzGerald GJ, Tarrant M, Aitken P, Fredriksen M, editors. Disaster Health Management: A Primer For Students And Practitioners. Abingdon, Oxon: Routledge, an imprint of the Taylor & Francis Group; 2017. p. 147–155.

6 Chan EYY. Public health humanitarian responses to natural disasters. Taylor & Francis; 2017.

7 Frumkin H, Hess J, Luber G, Malilay J, McGeehin M. Climate change: The public health response. *Am. J. Public Health* 2008; 98(3):435–445.

8 Watson KE, Singleton JA, Tippett V, Nissen LM. Defining pharmacists' roles in disasters: A Delphi study. *PLoS One* 2019; 14(12):e0227132.

9 Queensland Government. Queensland state disaster management plan: Reviewed May 2015: Disaster Management Act 2003. Brisbane: Queensland Disaster Management Committee; 2015.

10 Meagher J, Steinhardt R. Chapter 14: Preparedness. In: FitzGerald GJ, Tarrant M, Aitken P, Fredriksen M, editors. Disaster health management: A primer for students and practitioners. Abingdon, Oxon: Routledge, an imprint of the Taylor & Francis Group; 2017. p. 167–179.

11 Lonne B, McColl G, Marston G. Chapter 18: Community recovery. In: FitzGerald GJ, Tarrant M, Aitken P, Fredriksen M, editors. Disaster health management: A primer for students and practitioners. Abingdon, Oxon: Routledge, an imprint of the Taylor & Francis Group; 2017. p. 229–242.

# Part III

# Evidence and Stories from the Field

## Introduction

I do not want you to only take my word for it that pharmacists are vital to successful emergency response and have a valuable place in disaster and emergency management. So, in Part III of this book, I have provided evidence from the field with words from significant disaster health leaders and frontline disaster pharmacists. Together, they add another layer of credibility to this new field of study and provide valuable insight and opinions from the frontline of pharmacists in emergency management.

The next few chapters will take us on a journey through different themes that have emerged regarding pharmacists in disasters. Each theme includes several categories that were collated as part of a larger interview study that I conducted as part of my Ph.D. thesis. There were 28 interviews conducted with international stakeholders and experts in disaster health, pharmacy, and emergency management.

Additionally, I am honoured to introduce you to some of the incredible people that I have met that have helped shape my perspective in this field. The 'Stories from the Field' interviews were conducted before the COVID-19 pandemic was on the horizon and these participants have provided their consent to be named alongside their interview in this book. These 'Stories from the Field' interviews have been written as qualitative narratives which allow you as readers to become a part of the interview and to draw your own conclusions. It also provides insight into my thought processes while I was conducting the interviews.

DOI: 10.4324/b23292-10

# 8 Evidence from the Field: Disaster and Emergency Management Theme

## Introduction

The first theme we will review together is the overarching 'disaster and emergency management'. This theme ties to our earlier discussions in this book about emergency management more generally, the PPRR cycle, and the unique challenges faced by healthcare professionals in disasters and emergencies. While some of the content in this chapter may seem a little repetitive to our earlier discussions, they do present a different lens as it is not me saying that these things are important for you to know as a healthcare professional learning about emergency management but the 28 international key stakeholders that I interviewed who also agree that these are important aspects for pharmacists to know and understand. So, let's quickly revisit these important topics.

## Each Emergency Presents Unique Challenges

Disasters become public health emergencies quickly with the collapse of public health infrastructure and this will be highlighted again in Chapter 9 with the 'Story from the Field' interview with Dr. Fredrick (Skip) Burkle Jr., who is a well-respected senior international public health policy scholar. Additionally, the patient demographics of those adversely affected during a disaster or emergency are shifting. It is no longer solely acute injuries requiring care but exacerbations and management of people with chronic conditions. This is shown in the following comments from experienced disaster responders.

> There are so many people that have chronic diseases that if they're not managed it can make their life so intolerable. Yep, which also puts a strain on the disaster response system if it's not managed [A1][1]

> Hurricane Katrina we had millions of people displaced from their medications. Their pharmacies were gone, and these people were walking in and hadn't had their blood pressure medicine, their heart medicine, their diabetes medicine, for weeks. [19][1]

DOI: 10.4324/b23292-11

Another important aspect to pharmacists' key role in this, is the rules and regulations may need to extend beyond the disaster-impacted zone. Many of those adversely affected by disasters being evacuated or displaced, often leaving behind their prescriptions and medications and they are often evacuated outside of the disaster-impacted region for obvious reasons. However, when disaster-affected individuals are displaced and/or evacuated out of a disaster zone to a state which is not operating under the declared disaster rules, assisting them can be a challenge for health professionals. As the additional rules and regulations (i.e. extending emergency supplies and out-of-state licensing) are not usually in effect in a jurisdiction outside of the affected disaster zone.

Another aspect to consider with the changing patient demographic is catering for the patient's dietary needs, not just their medical wellbeing. In the event of a disaster, mass packages of food are usually provided by organisations to shelters and disaster-affected individuals, as their food supplies have been lost. The specific diets required by those with some chronic conditions is often not considered. Additionally, with the changes in pharmaceutical drug stock levels to smaller inventories kept in hospitals and pharmacies, small scale disasters can have a significant impact on a community if the supply chain of drugs is interrupted – even if only for a day or two.

While disasters and emergencies are unique and present different challenges for us, the healthcare system, and our communities to consider, there are also a lot of similarities as majority of disasters become a public health crisis and patients with chronic conditions need to be appropriately managed.

## Military and DMAT Objective in Emergencies

It's important to understand the broader purpose and objectives of medical support provided by the military and DMATs – Disaster Medical Assistance Teams. This helps us understand how they relate to pharmacists working in a disaster impacted region.

Acute injuries and illnesses are the primary focus of both the military and DMATs when heading into disaster zones. Something that I found interesting, was the objective of the military medical team when going on deployments is to treat their own if they get injured. Their pharmaceutical drug caches are not designed to tend to the needs of ongoing chronic conditions of the disaster-affected community. That's not to say that they don't assist in this way if asked to but that is not the purpose of their deployment. This is highlighted in the below quote by a military pharmacist and a disaster medical director.

*We don't send the whole hospital, but we tend to send small medical teams, generally to look after our own [people]. Especially when we're sending up a few hundred or a few thousand ... and of course, they're going to get cut, they're going to get hurt, they're moving heavy debris etc. That's when we've done that kind of health planning and say, well, what are our [soldiers] going to be dealing with and how are we going to keep them safe? How are we going to keep their hygiene levels up? How are we going to deal with all their cuts and scrapes etc.? That's our primary role, yes, to look after the military, whether it's our own or the coalition forces as well ... But certainly, it's difficult for us to treat chronic things so we don't necessarily deploy with diabetic drugs or Parkinson's drugs and stuff like that. We do very much acute care. [A6][1]*

*Usually we forget that, and we fail the challenge of not being able to provide for example treatment for chronic diseases or neglected cyst because we couldn't have the expertise of a pharmacist to analyse and plan what will happen the following month or years after the emergencies. [I4][1]*

The role of pharmacists in the military is almost completely logistics based – ensuring and maintaining the supply chain. While this is initially shocking to hear as a pharmacist, when you reflect on their primary purpose for deployment of the military medical team of acute injuries for the deployed soldiers, this does make some sense. This is outlined in the below quote from a military pharmacist.

*So, in the military, dare I say it, we are 95% logisticians, and 5% clinicians. Which is painful when you join the military after doing a five-year degree or four-year and one-year pre-reg [pre-registration], but I mean, at the end of the day it's absolutely crucial, and we're the ones who understand it the best. We're not dealing with blankets and boots, we're dealing with medical stores, which needs a completely different approach. [A6][1]*

Interestingly, it was also discussed that assistance during the response and recovery phases of a disaster should not be allowed to harm the local services. Local community pharmacies and clinicians cannot compete with the free services and medications provided by the military and DMAT services following a disaster. Thus, their deployments are intentionally kept short and addressing only the most pressing of acute issues. So, pharmacists working in this setting need to ensure emergency responses are minimising the potential risk of their and others' actions, putting into place risk mitigation strategies.

## Training and Skills Required in a Disaster

It is suggested being prepared for disasters and emergency management should be a part of every health professional's training. Unfortunately, the pharmacy perspective is often not included in generic disaster training for other professions and emergency management is often not covered in most pharmacy degrees or training. Those that I spoke to suggest, most pharmacists who work in disasters learn on the job from others with more experienced. The interviewees also discussed the need for better integration of pharmacists in emergency management and response teams. They emphasised that pharmacists need to be trained in all facets of emergency management to be adequately prepared and that they need to understand the role of other health professionals in disasters.

Additionally, there are identified challenges in finding adequate information on management of CBRN emergencies for pharmacists. There is a need to provide pharmacists with specific resources in treating and managing disaster specific injuries and illnesses as they are on the frontline of the health system and need to respond appropriately. Pharmacists need resources to help them identify the signs and symptoms of CBRN-affected individuals who present to pharmacies. This is discussed in the comments by an Australian hospital pharmacist and a US disaster pharmacist.

> ... So, now there's not a huge resource that's standardised across the country that the pharmacists can tap into when they're asked these clinical questions to give the answer. So, if we had a central repository of information to enable pharmacists to help with those clinical questions that would be really good. I contacted the eTGs [Australian electronic Therapeutic Guidelines] about that [previously available CBRN section] and they were unaware that people actually used it. So, that's why they took it out. [A9][1]

> ... when you think about the other possibilities which you really need to prepare for all the time, like nuclear, biological, chemical incidents and things like that, that information is really hard to find. At least good information about that is hard to find. [I9][1]

## Pharmacists as Translators

Currently, pharmacists are typically only included when the need for medications is considered during the response phase. One possible reason for this is in the difficulty that administration personnel face when deciding where pharmacists fit within disaster teams. As we previously discussed pharmacists don't neatly fit into any one category for administration to easily place or consider. Professionally, pharmacists' straddle across these multiple sectors including the logistics, medical, public health, and governance fields. They speak the different languages but not fully belonging to any of the individual sectors. This is highlighted in the comments made by an NGO pharmacist specific to emergency management:

> *Role of pharmacy was historically shared between a nurse and a logistician – taking that away from those positions. A nurse has many more roles that a pharmacist doesn't have and would be much more use as a nurse in these disasters setting and logisticians don't have the technical skills if something is a bit strange, while they can easily manage with the A-B and the setting up structures – they are not prescriptive in how things are set up. So, I see the key to be able to buffer between those types of positions. You [pharmacists] can speak medical to the medics and logistics to the logisticians, speaking the two languages. I think pharmacists are good at changing their language depending on who they are speaking to, even with the same information ... It's treading between the medical teams and the logistics team and you're [pharmacists] are essentially not in either but more under the logistical head – how to be in those discussions takes a lot of diplomacy, trying to get the fridge operating at the right temperature or why we need air-conditioning for the drugs. It's probably the least of the head of logistics concern in the scheme of things. [A13]*[1]

Additionally, pharmacists also work across both the medical and public health sectors looking after the welfare of patients and the community in everyday circumstances and in times of emergencies. Many patients tend to seek out pharmacists for public health advice in community pharmacies before considering making an appointment with another healthcare professional or going to overcrowded hospitals. The recognition of the value pharmacists provides with regards to the health needs in a community during everyday circumstances and in times of crisis are highlighted in the quote by an Australian emergency manager.

**[Everyday]**

> *We have pharmacies open seven days a week. So, [they] wouldn't be open seven days a week if there wasn't a need for that. There must be enough need to generate the income. So, the more I think about it, the more I'm thinking how important the bloody pharmacist is. I've never thought about that. It's stressing me out! But even in my little rural community, when I'm out at the farm, that pharmacy is open seven days a week. It might only be for two hours on a Sunday morning, but he's open seven days. You go, wow, I never thought about that, but, yeah, there must be a need.*

[Crisis]

> *Part of the challenge is actually integrating or liaising with the disaster welfare aspects of a disaster, who are more people focused [and that] is probably where the pharmacist is going to get greater understanding of their role. So, I think that in the health setting, what I'm seeing in Australia and in New Zealand, public health people have a different mindset to the medical people or primary healthcare. So, the idea of holistic medical – this is going to upset doctors, but doctors are very much, come in, fix this problem, I go out. Probably such souls having a close connection to the hospital/ambulance system. But I think that the pharmacist is more about people and probably has that more affinity to the psychosocial welfare aspects of disasters. [A1]*[1]

The problem with attempting to achieve a role change in emergency management is that such changes need to be thought of and enacted before a disaster event occurs. The status quo tends to be maintained by default when chaos ensues. Once a disaster or emergency happens, it is too late to change pharmacists' roles and introduce new areas that pharmacists can contribute to. This is highlighted in the following quote from an emergency manager.

> *The hardest time to do it is when something's happening because people are not open to new ideas. So, the idea's got to be done through the lead up to an [emergency] event. [A1]*[1]

There is a struggle to keep the momentum following a disaster to carry through pharmacists' role changes as people tend to lose interest as time passes after the emergency. This is when there is potential for pharmacists' roles to be lost or dropped as memories of pharmacists' contributions dim and interest in preparing for disasters exponentially dips.

## Chapter Reference

1 Watson KE The Roles of Pharmacists in Disaster Health Management in Natural and Anthropogenic Disasters. [Thesis]. QUT ePrints: Queensland University of Technology; 2019 Available from: https://eprints.qut.edu.au/130757/.

# 9 Story from the Field: An Interview with Dr. Fredrick (Skip) Burkle Jr.

## Introduction

I am honoured to introduce you to some of the incredible people that I have met that have helped shape my perspective in this field. The 'Stories from the Field' interviews were conducted before the COVID-19 pandemic was on the horizon and these participants have provided their consent to be named along with their interview in this book. Dr. Frederick M. (Skip) Burkle Jr. is a well respected senior international public policy scholar. Dr. Burkle, Jr. is an American physician known for his work in disaster and emergency response and humanitarian assistance, public health preparedness, human rights, international diplomacy, and peacekeeping.[1] Dr. Burkle, Jr. provides a unique perspective from a historical and systems thinking lens about pharmacists' roles in disasters and emergencies.

To start the interview, we discussed some small talk about the recent World Association for Disaster and Emergency Medicine (WADEM) congresses that I attended in Brisbane, Australia in 2018 and Toronto, Canada in 2016. WADEM had recently announced that the Global Leadership in Emergency Public Health Award would be named in honour of Dr. Burkle Jr., recognising his outstanding contributions to the science and practice of humanitarian relief efforts. *I started the recording and go through my prepared spiel on providing verbal informed consent to record the interview.* "Thank you for taking the time for this interview, I am honoured to be speaking with you today. Please share your honest thoughts, opinions, and perspective about pharmacists' roles in disasters and emergencies". *I say, hoping to build rapport across the phone. I really want to know what he honestly thinks, and I hope I'm prepared to hear the answer. In my mind, I chide myself again for jumping to the assumption that pharmacists have a place in emergency management and remind myself that the research needs to speak for itself. I can't wish it to be so.*

"Dr. Burkle, Jr. could you please tell me about your profession?" *I say as clearly as I can, silently berating myself for speaking too fast during the consent spiel and telling myself to pace my voice, not everyone can*

DOI: 10.4324/b23292-12

*understand the Australian accent, our colloquialisms, or the speed at which I talk.* "I am a physician, an educator, and a researcher - scientist. I am a senior fellow and scientist at the Harvard Humanitarian Initiative of Harvard University at Harvard School of Public Health. I am also a senior international public policy scholar at the Woodrow Wilson Centre for International Scholars in Washington, D.C". *Dr. Burkle Jr. says and asks me to call him Skip. I muse to myself that he has a great pace of voice. Contemplative but assured, I am struck with a sense of the wealth of knowledge and experience he has that I am about to become privy to.*

### Dr. Burkle Jr.'s Disaster Experience

"What is your experience in dealing with unpredictable events or disasters?" *I probe.* "Well, that has been my lifelong career. Primarily I have dealt with complex humanitarian emergencies in war. So, I have been in six major wars and over 40 complex emergencies. I've done research on natural disasters, but I have not personally responded to them. I teach disaster medicine and humanitarian assistance. I've taught it at several venues but I'm also one of the organisers of the first courses that has been given internationally to healthcare providers. I am 77 years of age, so I've been around for a while, when there were only a handful of us - disaster health experts. Our legacy has been to produce more people that are well trained to provide disaster management and humanitarian assistance. So that's essentially what I've done. That's what I'm known for". *Skip states. I experience two emotions while Skip is outlining his experience, firstly – I should have done more homework on who I was interviewing and had more intelligent questions to ask and secondly, wow! I am so fortunate that I've had the opportunity to speak to Skip and get his perspective on this topic of pharmacists and emergencies.*

"What kind of health professionals do you train?" *I ask.* "Good question. Well, I'm a retired navy captain and I was called up for five different wars. I was also the first minister of health in Iraq. So, I've trained a lot of military people. But also, obviously civilians that would work in NGOs. I'm on the board of directors of International Rescue Committee which is the world's largest refugee NGO. I'm also part of the advisory board for the Red Cross. So, I've pretty much worked for and trained people from all of those venues - NGOs, military, Red Cross and probably a few others. They're pretty much across the board. Most of our training includes multidisciplinary and interprofessional students". *Skip responds.*

### Dr. Burkle Jr.'s Experience with Pharmacists

"Have you come across pharmacists in your various roles?" *I ask feeling subconscious and holding my breath.* "Yes. Interesting ... I don't recall many pharmacists at all in the courses except for the military ones in my day but I have worked with pharmacists ... but pharmacists at least in the humanitarian training programs are getting more and more popular and more and more depended on". *Skip recounts and then pauses as if retrieving a memory.* "I think one of the issues - I had to think back in preparation for this discussion - **when I was first drafted in the Vietnam war in 1968 and went to a forward casualty receiving facility with the United States Marines, it's meatball surgery - lots of corpsmen and doctors. We had no nurses. But I remember a pharmacist. There was just one. The guy worked his tail off.** But our unit because it was so close to North Vietnam, kept getting hit by artillery from the north. So, we still saw our own casualties, but they changed it to a children's hospital. With that change in patient population, the supply chain for the military changed dramatically. So, I had to work with the pharmacist a lot. It was a humanitarian kind of partnership". *Skip stops and switches back to the present,* "Everybody now depends on pharmacists especially with the NGOs that go off to places whether it's Nepal or Haiti or Syria or any other place; whether it's a natural disaster and public health emergency of international concern like Ebola or a complex humanitarian emergency/ war. **The demands for pharmacists are tremendous** ... pharmacists are worth their weight in gold. They and the logisticians work hand in hand – they are some of the most talented and heavily relied upon".

*I start to respond but realise that Skip has more to say on the topic, so I go quiet again.* "**I think the problem in the past was that pharmacists were quietly working all the time, and everybody just depended on them. They never seemed to complain.** I don't remember them complaining like everybody else did in the military, because they had so much work to do in keeping the supplies going. So that is a big factor. **I've never been in a situation where any pharmacist let me down. That's for sure.** I mean maybe we just focused in on physicians do this and nurses do that. But nowadays it's becoming more multidisciplinary. So, the pharmacists are coming out of the woodwork to take the usual courses like the health course - health emergencies in large populations or the ones from the NGOs and things like that, that previously were just for physicians and nurses. As we get more multidisciplinary, we have a greater body of lectures and a more diverse student body. I have no doubt that if pharmacists are not already giving some lectures, they should be giving lectures tied to the whole logistics issues and probably what we'd call vulnerable populations. What are the pharmaceutical requirements for children, elderly, women, the disabled, to understand the medications? In a sense the pharmacists are also logisticians. They really are. So, it's I think the change I would say, even reminding me from my earlier conversation today, is that the pharmacists are coming out of the woodwork". *I wonder if pharmacists are really doing these lectures and are sought after by NGOs. I write a mental note to ask others of their experiences.*

## Where Do Pharmacists' Fit in the PPRR Cycle

*I look down at my list of interview questions, trying to think where to go to next in this interview.* "Where in the emergency management PPRR cycle do you believe the pharmacists have these roles?" *I ask.* "Excellent question. I'll give you a high mark for that one. I think one of the things is, we in the field have always been response oriented. So, everything is response, response, response. Well, I've been one of the ones that authored a number of articles about the public health. **Most of these disasters, if not all of them, turn out in a very short period of time to be public health emergencies or within two weeks become a public health emergency.** Over a long period of time, **90% of the deaths and morbidity are actually from public health infrastructure loss, not from the war and weapons or direct disaster impacts.** But every single disaster in a very short period of time when the public health infrastructure gets destroyed or is no longer functional, then a bunch of public health preventable diseases (e.g. diarrhoea, respiratory illnesses) come out".

"**The pharmacists become part of the screening process in managing these preventable public health diseases.** Over the last decade we've moved away from solely focusing on response and broadening to the entire PPRR cycle, so working on prevention, preparedness, response, and recovery/rehabilitation. **For every $1 you spend in prevention and preparedness you save $4 in response.** It's just going to get too darned expensive to only focus on response". *Skip replies and continues.*

"In terms of pharmacy, what does this translate to? Will there be drug kits? What form will they take? What role will pharmacists have in setting up, designing, or managing these kits? How do you design kits to cater to these community non-communicable needs? How do you mobilise it? Physicians and nurses can't do it themselves because that's a knowledge base that we don't know that much about, but pharmacists are experts in medication management. **Pharmacists know something about the community in terms of women, children, elderly, the vulnerable populations and then from that you can extrapolate the non-communicable diseases and what the risk would be for that population during a disaster or public health emergency.** One of the things with Hurricane Katrina that was known - I wrote an editorial on this particular article that came out about it.[2] The article is really very important in the fact that all the Red Cross nurses that were running the shelters - were not at all prepared for the public health consequences that their residents began to have. They didn't know how to really deal with people coughing and having diarrhoea and things like that. They were more trauma oriented or acute care. So that was a big concern. People weren't necessarily prepared for it. Everybody can make the case that the more we put into prevention and preparedness the more you're going to save in response. Pharmacists and pharmacy organizations have to be aware of that". "That's a really interesting point".

*I mention and make a note to learn more about the PPRR cycle and where and how pharmacists fit.*

*Skip muses,* "You know, in Australia, you have the prepared community concepts. We don't have them in the United States. I think it's really good idea. Whereas, in the United States, each state is sort of in charge of their own disaster planning. So, when something happens in a community in the United States a bunch of generic stuff gets sent to it as a first response and it is often not what is needed by that community - It's wasted. But the prepared community concept that Australia has, turns that responsibility for disaster planning, prevention, and preparedness to the community level and not the state level. **It's effective because it is recognised that each community is discrete and unique.** If you allow the leaders of the community to develop the disaster plan it would be more specific in terms of what they need based on geography or population density or the most common issues. Then that information goes to a disaster bank which is at the state level. So, when the disaster happens in that community, assistance isn't delayed by sending assessment teams to find out what the community needs. They just trust what was done in that community's planning and immediately your state sends all those supplies that they have in the disaster bank, to that specific community. What the studies have shown is that with that both the response and the rehabilitation at the community level were much faster and more efficient". *Skip concludes and I wonder if pharmacists are involved at the community level to help with the disaster planning from a health perspective.*

## Pharmacists' Roles in Disasters – Logistics or Clinical or Both?

"Wow, that's so interesting, thank you for sharing it with me". *I gush thinking of future avenues I might want to explore. I shake myself back to the present interview,* "From your experience, do you see the role of pharmacists still being based solely in that logistics and supply chain management? Or do you think there is capacity for pharmacists to be more involved, say in clinical aspects of emergency management?" *I state, feeling like I'm on the right track with my interviewing when Skip excitedly replies,* "Yeah, I'm glad you brought that up. Very definitely the latter, **pharmacists have more roles in disasters than just logistics**. However, previously pharmacists and it may be the culture - they stand behind the counter in the pharmacies and pretty much there was no conversation or interaction. But over the years they have become much more engaged in giving education to patients and now they give shots for flu and other clinical services. So, you can have a real engaged conversation with them about disease. Again because of my age, the pharmacists I knew back in the day were "just pill pushers". If you asked them something, they'd either have to look it up or say I don't know. Now you can have an engaged and intellectual conversation with pharmacists about side effects and treatment options. More broadly and especially in the humanitarian field - pharmacists do have to know a hell of a lot more than just prescription process - fill it, give it, tell the side effects. **They engage with us clinically when we are running out of supplies or we're looking for alternative treatment options**. For example, I had to manage the largest Bubonic Plague epidemic in Vietnam. One of the things about Yersinia Pestis which is the bacteria that causes Plague, it is one of the bacteria that is able to build up resistance to antibiotics in no time flat. So, at that time I only had four or five antibiotics available to me. That's when I talked to the pharmacist and asked, hey what can you get me? So, I'd say they are becoming more and more part of the clinical team. **I mean everybody that I talk to says pharmacists are an important part of their team**". *Skip recounts and continues.* "Actually, the one organization I work with before I deploy is the WHO. They keep a current list of the medications that all countries have available – the essential medicines list.[3] Many of the medications in poorer countries are ones we used in the West decades ago - specifically mental health medications. Pharmacists are rare in the field, and one usually works with nurses in stabilising patients from the available list of medications. But I have been in refugee camps where many suffer mental illnesses, some situational, some organic. One has to assess these issues quickly. The first thing I look at are a list of pharmaceuticals normally used for mental health issues in that country such a manic-depressive disease or schizophrenia or severe depression. In refugee camps, one has to restart the medications rapidly to stabilise the patients whether they are experience cardiac, respiratory, infectious diseases or mental health challenges. **We feel lucky if we have a pharmacist on the team**. Some aid workers come with their own medications but if these medications are used there are often too many side effects and the local practitioners who are nurses, not physicians, are not familiar with them and their side effects. Once the aid workers leave so go the new medications so one has to know the pharmacopeia of every country before one deploys. Its probably one of the most critical duties pharmacists and physicians have".[4]

## Disaster Health and Pharmacists' Scope of Practice

*I'm a little nervous but probe a little further and ask,* "Following on from that, do you believe assisting in disasters is within the current scope or practice of a pharmacist?" *Skip replies,* "**Oh God yes or it should be! I have talked to pharmacists in the past and suggested that they write down their experiences and publish them in journals**. I'm not sure whether they ever did. This was during the SARS epidemic. What we asked them to do was to write some articles about how the pharmacists and the pharmacies gear up for natural disasters and public health emergencies of international concern which are the infectious diseases - things whether it be SARS, Ebola, or Zika. **If this information is written down, these pharmacists become teachers for other pharmacists to learn from their experience.** More and more clinicians are looking to find out what are the different treatment options. What are the polypharmacy issues when you start adding and mixing in new medications? Those are the things that we as physicians want to discuss with the pharmacist. There are standards, for example the sphere concept in humanitarian assistance.[5] I'd be interested and would have to look it up and see whether they have any standards regarding pharmacy. But if they don't, they may in the future when updated standards are published. Maybe you can answer that for me? But there should be sphere standards for pharmaceuticals written by the International Committee of the Red Cross (ICRC) and WHO so that we know exactly what's there. We're getting so specific that we can tie medications to the disaster event (e.g. what are the most common ones?)" *Skip states.*

*He pauses and I can hear he takes a sip of water before continuing,* "When Ebola happened, I remember being on the phones with Geneva in the early morning hours here in Hawaii, US. They were saying, we need more emergency physicians. Can you send them? I said, wait a second this is a public health emergency. Emergency physicians don't necessarily know a lot about public health. So, we talked about that. As a matter of fact, they ended up writing an article about the lack of public health skills being the Achilles heel.[6] So many people that responded to Ebola in West Africa had to relearn an awful lot". *Skip pauses for a moment and continues,* "I'm sure the pharmaceutical issues with that were amazingly complex. A lot of them are simply because the public health infrastructure is gone or destroyed, and medications are required. There is research out of New Orleans after Hurricane Katrina. I remember reading the data - people showing up to the different clinics or evacuation centres because their homes were destroyed. **The percentage that had showed up with some medication, or others that did not, many were pregnant, or had chronic conditions - it mirrored society. It was amazing not only how many people needed their medication right away or stated that they did or did not know what medications they were on. Sometimes the pharmacist had to play tag with them to reconcile the patient's medications -** what size was it? What are you taking it for? Any information we could get on their usual medications or allergies. **So, pharmacists are an important part of that educational team. There's no doubt about that, no doubt about it at all**". *There's silence in the call, as I take in all the information and begin trying to process it in my mind - pharmacists are valuable in disasters.*

## Specific Pharmacists' Roles

*I begin explaining what some of the literature states about previous pharmacists' roles in disasters and I ask Skip's thoughts on the pharmacists' role in managing non-communicable or chronic conditions. He responds,* "Since non-communicable diseases are increasing and more and more of the larger percentage of disaster-affected individuals require chronic disease care - this is not something that the doctors and nurses want to deal with. They want to deal with the blood and guts. **I don't think I'm wrong in saying this - my prediction is that nobody will want to do it. They'll say, kick it to the pharmacist**". *It's an interesting thought that perhaps some of the pharmacists' roles in disasters are backfilling non-urgent roles (e.g. prescribing and managing chronic conditions) to free up others to manage the acute and immediate injuries.* "What about pharmacists prescribing and administering vaccinations?" *I ask.* "Well, they already do that. It's a public service, **it's easier to go to the pharmacy than to go to the doctor's office**. Especially if a prolonged disaster or if there's an outbreak of some sort". *Skip responds.*

## Pharmacists' Roles Need to be Known

"Are there any roles pharmacists should or shouldn't do or why they could do a role but shouldn't?" *I ask, taking a sip of water.* "Well, they should do it as part of a team. Whenever they are doing different roles or it's a decision that's made at some level everybody in the disaster team needs to know that it is part of the pharmacist's responsibility and it's okay. **If a disaster happens and pharmacists are part of some kind of response and the other team members don't know what they are doing or what their role is, then whatever pharmacists have done in preparation doesn't mean diddly-squat** *[aka doesn't mean anything]*. It's got to be known by the broader disaster health team and response. You can't after the fact say, oh okay, oh so you have this training and could have helped in x, y, or z. I mean there's got to be some mechanism of understanding. Trespassing the professional boundaries is what's really difficult. There's got to be some mechanism where whatever training there is with the pharmacist it's known and is also included as part of the training and knowledge of others - nurses, physicians, etc. Finding out about the potential roles' pharmacists could assist with during a disaster cancels out a lot of the benefits as it needs to be implemented in the planning and preparedness. The other important thing is pharmacists' medicine mitigation because they can take a tremendous amount of the strain away from those that might be dealing with acute issues. Not that they don't also deal with acute issues. **But it's important that chronic or non-communicable issues are dealt with as there's not much time before these issues would become acute if not treated/given medication. That's where the**

**pharmacists' prevention roles really come in**. Our usual design of disaster teams doesn't really cater for low-acuity and non-communicable issues. So that would be the kind of clinical role that I'd see the pharmacist taking, especially in non-communicable disease, the chronic conditions - the kidney problems, the respiratory problems, the diabetes, etc. The one measure of that is how many of those patients are prevented from coming into the acute situation". *Skip responds.*

## Barriers to Pharmacists' Roles in Disasters

"What do you see as the barriers to implementing these types of roles that we've discussed in the preparedness phase for the next disaster?" *I ask.* "I guess, the barriers are - territory. Pharmacists do this. Nurses do that. It's always been that kind of thing with healthcare. I think that the younger generation of healthcare providers are less territorial. But that depends a lot on where you are practicing. As I alluded to before, I never previously relied on a pharmacist for a lot of education. I always thought I knew more about the drugs than they did. Basically, they filled the prescriptions and said very little. That has totally changed. That has totally changed! **They're the experts now**. Probably sometime slowly in my own life I overcame it and started seeing pharmacists more and more as colleagues that I can chat about a disease situation. We're much more collegial. That has been a big, big change! That should positively transmit to a disaster situation". *Skip replies. I am excited to hear pharmacists are being taken seriously in disasters, granted it's more of a recent shift than I would have perhaps thought it should be but at least there is progress, and pharmacists are being recognised for our unique contributions to disasters.*

"What suggestions do you have for an alternative or better implementation of pharmacists into disaster health management?" *I question.* "Well first off - they've got to become a legitimate team member. I don't know how my physician colleagues will respond to that. But they would probably say, **well I can see they have to be but right now they're not. You've got to get the acknowledgement that they are part of the team.** Everybody responds to that. So, whatever it takes to get that. **Getting the training, broad-based – pharmacists need to have broad-based training, not just pharmacy specific. But they need to understand the problems that everybody has at each level of the disaster care model.** Then a big thing would be to start their own pharmaceutical disaster training programs for other pharmacists. Out of that will be just like what happened decades ago in medicine. That is, you'll get the doers and the people that want to just respond like that and those that are more interested in prevention and preparedness and those that are really damn good teachers. Then you become more value-added to the team approach, the multidisciplinary team approach". *Skip responds.*

## Summing Up

"Skip, thank you for your time I have really enjoyed speaking with you and learning from your insight. It was important to me to include different perspectives outside of pharmacists in this research study. I want to know from disaster health experts like yourself, whether there is a place in disasters for pharmacists and if so, what their roles might be. Is there anything else you'd like to add?" *I say, hoping my sincere gratitude for this interview is conveyed in my voice. Skip responds,* "I congratulate you on what you're doing. I hesitated initially because for all the things I've done in the field - it was just trying to get anything off the ground. But things have changed a lot. Now is the time for what you're doing to be a major component. That question - are pharmacists an essential part of disasters or could they be? you're asking two questions there. I think at this stage of the game the majority of people from medicine and probably nursing - they would answer the first part - are pharmacists currently essential members - they would probably say no. But then you asked, but could or should pharmacists be essential members? My colleagues would probably universally say 100% yes. **So, it's just the fact that pharmacists are just not part of that broader team concept yet**, maybe in some instances, especially if you get people who are sort of thinking after you ask the question. *They're not now but boy yes, they should be!*

## Chapter References

1 Smith E, Burkle F. Interview with Professor Frederick M. *"Skip" Burkle, Jr.* 2018. https://wadem.org/wp-content/uploads/2018/05/interview-with-professor-frederick-burkle-jr.pdf
2 Burkle FM. Sheltering the sheltered: Protecting the public health and educating the workforce. *Prehosp. Disaster Med.* 2009; 24:506–507.
3 World Health Organization. *WHO model list of essential medicines* 20th Edition. World Health Organization; 2017.
4 Van Ommeren M. Protecting the most vulnerable: Supporting people with mental disorders during disasters. Devex; 2016 [cited 2021 Jan 3]; Available from: https://www.devex.com/news/protecting-the-most-vulnerable-supporting-people-with-mental-disorders-during-disasters-88149
5 Sphere P. *The Sphere project: Humanitarian charter and minimum standards in humanitarian response.* U.K.: Practical Action Publishing [distributor]; 2011.
6 Burkle Jr. FM. Operationalizing public health skills to resource poor settings: Is this the Achilles heel in the Ebola epidemic campaign? *Dis. Med. Public Health Preparedness* 2015; 9(1):44–46.

# 10 Evidence from the Field: Community Theme

## Introduction

The second theme we will review together is the overarching theme of 'community'. This theme highlights the important role that pharmacists and pharmacies have within their communities both for disaster-affected individuals as well as other first responders (e.g., deployed search and rescue teams, other healthcare workers, etc.). People rely on their pharmacists to continue to be accessible and maintain pharmacy operations (e.g., medications, reliable information, etc.). While some of the content in this chapter may seem a little repetitive to our earlier discussions, they do present a different lens as these are the words of others working in the field with extensive disaster and emergency expertise. So, let's quickly revisit these important topics.

## Emergency Plans

Emergency and disaster planning need to be included in pharmacies' emergency or BCPs. This acknowledges that there is an inevitability of a disaster or emergency affecting pharmacies like any other organisation and outlines the management strategies they plan to employ and action to handle the emergency. A BCP assists organisations (e.g., pharmacies, clinics, etc.) in planning and preparing for immediate and long-term response and recovery activities to emergencies. It outlines the actions necessary to ensure continuance of patient care and operations. Pharmacies are no exception from needing to have a BCP. A government disaster manager illustrates the dilemma faced by pharmacies in disasters and how they need to have a BCP as they have a duty of care:

> ... there's an obligation that's part of the business continuity to make a decision that you're going to be there for that community hell or high water. But how are you going to manage it? [I13][1]

DOI: 10.4324/b23292-13

Disaster management plans are especially important for pharmacies which are often found in potential disaster-prone areas and provide care to those individuals in the community who are more vulnerable to adverse health outcomes in a disaster. This was highlighted in a story of a national disaster simulated exercise described by this government disaster manager.

> *I'll give you an example – so we did the national exercise based on a relatively close tsunami event affecting the coast … As part of that – the majority of the coast lines would be affected and there'd be little warning because unfortunately it was a close tsunami … The climate there is in fact lovely, it's beautiful – and it's where a lot of people come to retire. They come to the sea and the beach and so they build a lot of retirement villages and homes there and of course that means you have an elderly population quite close to the beach. As a consequence and a fact of life is, GP practices and pharmacies are attracted to those sorts of populations because there is a need. So, they build their premises in the same sort of locations which are adjacent to these retirement villages and retirement homes and unfortunately because majority is a sweeping statement – but majority – older people like to have flat surfaces to walk along – flat surfaces and beaches, tsunamis love. So basically, when we did the mapping for all the inundation zones and we looked at it and overlayed it where the pharmacies and GP practices were, I think there were probably 2 out of the 20 that were not lined to be inundated with the tsunami wave. So, I would suggest to you, that there's possibly 18 pharmacies that aren't going to be applying their trade for a considerable time even if they have got some form of business fall back plan, because as you know pharmacies have to be licenced premise and there's a raft of legislation around securing capabilities there, double locks and controlled drugs, etc.*
>
> *So, none of it's easy, but I don't know how much attention is paid to what one would do if that scenario happened. The impact for the community I would suggest would be huge for that sort of loss. So yeah, does that sort of give an indication of why I am a little concerned – I think probably on the domestic front, I'm not sure that enough attention is paid to what either their [pharmacy's] business continuity plan would be because I don't know if it's looked at in as much depth as it could be. [I13]*[1]

Alternatively, if a disaster inundates a pharmacy infrastructure that does not necessarily mean the pharmacy services and the pharmacist's expertise are rendered unavailable. With adequate preparedness and a comprehensive BCP, pharmacists can continue to provide services to their communities under difficult circumstances. Hurricane Andrew in

1992 wiped out almost every pharmacy building in Miami, United States; however, the local pharmacists continued to provide an essential service to their community for months after the hurricane had passed. This was mentioned by a US pharmacist.

> *Another great example is when [Hurricane] Andrew came through in 1992 at Miami. The extended recovery phase for a pharmacist down there was significant because basically every pharmacy in Miami got the windows blown out and all the stock destroyed. They had to bring in basically tractor trailers and set up temporary pharmacies on the parking lots of places where there used to be actual pharmacies. The pharmacists that worked in those had to basically work through that recovery period until such time as their infrastructure was back in place. That was an extended period of time, sometimes months before everyone was back to normal. [I5]*[1]

A business cannot rely on the tacit, corporate knowledge of their experienced staff who may have weathered previous events or lived in disaster-prone areas for years. If this knowledge is not recorded or embedded in the pharmacy's BCP, the pharmacy's ability to prepare or respond to future disasters may be impacted. The reason BCPs are so important for pharmacies taking an all-hazard approach to disasters is because of the strong reliance on the important role pharmacists and pharmacies have in their communities. So, it's not just our pharmacies that need a BCP but we as pharmacists need to have our own personal and professional emergency plan. Are you prepared to go to work if you are not scheduled but a disaster occurs? Have you considered balancing family obligations with work and professional obligations during an emergency?

## Importance of Pharmacy in the Community

Pharmacy services are relied upon not only by those disaster-affected individuals but also by those volunteer and workers who come into the disaster-affected zones to assist as highlighted by an incident command controller.

> *So, I think that pharmacists have an important role in supporting first response, even in terms of like I've seen some bushfires where there'll be 200 firefighters in and the first thing you spend the first few days going to the pharmacist getting stuff for them, because they've left it all back in their home state. [A1]*[1]

It was identified in the interviews that a pharmacy is a community landmark or hub of the community. Pharmacists are identified as the third largest group of healthcare professionals and are the most accessible – being the most widely distributed healthcare profession in a community. Pharmacies are more accessible than supermarkets, banks, or medical centres.[2] So, it's easy to see why pharmacists are a significant asset that could be utilised in disaster and emergency management. This was highlighted by an US pharmacist:

> *The other thing that makes pharmacists uniquely well suited for disaster response is just the sheer number, at least in the United States, I'm not as familiar with other countries and how they're set up, but in the United States we have over 60,000 community pharmacies and the average distance that a patient live from a community pharmacy, if they live in a city, is less than a mile. If they live in a rural area, it's typically somewhere between five and 10 miles to the closest pharmacy. That's a greater density than any other healthcare provider. [16]*

Pharmacists are often operating as first responders in a disaster as those adversely affected by a disaster come to pharmacies as their first port of call to get help. Thus, community members and governments expect pharmacists to keep pharmacies open and to provide pharmacy services. This is highlighted in the quote from an Australian community pharmacist from their experience working in a cyclone.

> *A lot of the doctors weren't open or available. The hospital was chock-a-block [Australian slang for crammed full], so there was certainly an immense amount of primary care. I can't remember how many cuts, injuries I saw that day that I either literally treated myself or bandaged up or referred to the hospital, if I felt it was necessary. So, there was certainly a lot more primary care stuff, rather than your traditional dispensing ... definitely the role becomes more of a primary care, nursing, first aid type role in the immediate aftermath. [A12][1]*

Disaster healthcare professionals mentioned how vital the community pharmacy is in acting as a communication hub and surveillance tool in the recovery of the local community. Often it was the community pharmacy which would be the first business to be operational following a disaster event as discussed by this US disaster emergency responder. So, the roles of pharmacists in the community are vitally important and they are the litmus test to indicate the recovery of the community. Pharmacists are not just relied on for their pharmacy services but also for their fundamental role in the community and providing public health and primary care.

## Chapter References

1 Watson KE. *The roles of pharmacists in disaster health management in natural and anthropogenic disasters*. [Thesis]. QUT ePrints: Queensland University of Technology; 2019. Available from: https://eprints.qut.edu.au/130757/

2 The Pharmacy Guild of Australia. *Submission in response to the competition policy review draft report*. National Secretariat, Barton, ACT; 2014.

# 11 Story from the Field: An Interview with Dr. Robert Dunne

## Introduction

Let's meet another of the incredible people that I have met that have helped shape my perspective in this field that makes up our 'Stories from the Field'. Dr Robert Dunne is a emergency physician with a Disaster Medical Assistance Team (DMAT) and has worked alongside pharmacists while responding to emergencies and disasters. Dr. Dunne provides insight into the DMAT set-up and the commitment to having strong pharmacy representation. Reminder that these interviews were conducted before the COVID-19 pandemic was on the horizon and these participants have provided their consent to be named along with their interview in this book.

"Thank you for agreeing to participate in this interview on pharmacists' roles in disasters, can you tell me about your experiences working in disasters?" *I begin.* "I have been involved in a federal disaster response team - what's called a disaster medical assistance team (DMAT) as an emergency physician - since 1997. I also have served in a planning and response capacity locally for my hospital". *Dr. Dunne responds.* "What kind of roles are required of you during these disaster events?" *I continue.* "Generally, I serve as a medical officer, doing medical care, working shifts. I have, on a couple of occasions, served in a coordination role". *Robert replies.*

"Would you say that you were fully equipped with your training and skills to handle the challenging circumstances of those types of events?" *I ask, wondering if the training is comprehensive for the medical profession.* "Not completely. It is something that's part of the curriculum for emergency physician training, but it's not a very big part of the curriculum. Then, when you join these teams, there's some very basic orientation and safety training but, mostly, you end up learning by being deployed with people who have done it more and have had experience. The first few times you're out, your kind of learning as you go. You're not really completely trained to go do it when you first do it". *Robert recounts. It makes me wonder if perhaps the same would be true of other*

DOI: 10.4324/b23292-14

*healthcare professions and how much can be taught in a classroom before being deployed.*

## DMAT Set-Up

"Where do you think pharmacists fit or what role do pharmacists have in disaster health management?" *I question.* "Let's take a moment and just talk about the federal team set-up. There's always been a big commitment by pharmacists and to pharmacists. **Pharmacists have always been considered an essential team position.** The basic response element of these teams is the 35-person team. That includes two pharmacists. Your team is not complete to be deployed unless you have at least two pharmacists. Sometimes we'll actually share pharmacists between teams if a team doesn't have a pharmacist available. **Pharmacists have always been deemed essential, for a variety of reasons.** One is medicine management. There's a very large drug cache that gets deployed with the teams: literally two pallet loads of drugs, plus another partial pallet of refrigerated ones that'll go with the team. The pharmacist has got control over the inventory and they need to have knowledge on how the drugs are used to provide support to the physicians for prescribing. Then they have to track the drug use so that we can get resupply for the right things as needed. In addition, a number of years ago now, we moved to using an electronic medical record, even for disaster deployments. It's a very simple and kind of similar to what maybe an ambulance uses, but a fairly simple electronic record that actually has some order entry on that so the pharmacist can track a little bit more of what's going on in real time. This was nice on the command side because then the pharmacist who's supervising the overall response - maybe even remotely in terms of inventory management - could monitor what's being used to try and move things forward to the disaster deployment a little bit more quickly. **In my personal experience on our team, our pharmacists are great. Having a pharmacist when you're using unfamiliar medications is really, really helpful".** *Robert pauses.*

## Pharmacists' Skills

*I wait a moment before moving on as I get the impression Dr. Dunne is between thoughts. Robert continues,* "I think pharmacists are really essential. One of the things that we see a lot after disasters is, we see a population that's more severely affected because they have a lot of mental illnesses. Often, these people are on fairly complicated medical regimens, and having a pharmacist to work with especially given some of these things may be things that I don't typically prescribe, or even maybe don't see that often, even in my regular emergency medicine practice. The pharmacists can give me a lot of information on what might be a substitution if we're in an austere situation and that person is on - particularly some of the psychiatric medicine that we had a lot of patients on after Hurricane Katrina; what would be a substitute for that. I mean the pharmacy role is incredible, as well as the fact that pharmacists are very familiar with the best way to manage and store medications, something that physicians aren't really going to know. Some things say that you have to refrigerate them, but could they actually tolerate not being refrigerated for, say, 30 days? For a two-week deployment, that may be fine. Other things that refrigeration may be a bit more important for stability, that's something that's going to be a little out of a lot of physicians' experiences. The same thing with dilution and augmentation of drugs, that's something that I don't do a lot. I mean occasionally, when the emergency department is really busy, I may end up doing something like that, but in a disaster situation that level of knowledge is really important because we still want to avoid making things worse. We want to avoid medical and medication errors in the disaster situation. The other thing I saw - particularly in Haiti - where we had a lot of paediatrics, and a lot of paediatric critical care is about paediatric drug dosing. Pharmacists were very helpful and supportive for that".

## Pharmacists as DMAT members

"What kind of roles do your pharmacists have on your DMATs?" *I enquire, wondering if I will hear the classic response of logistics and supply chain management.* "They're in a planning role. Every team participates in the drug cache development. We track what we've actually used through model simulations. Then we look at typical emergency department utilisation of drugs to make sure we're actually bringing the right equipment. That's one thing that our pharmacists all participate in, is creating of the drug cache, but also in putting together after-action reports and then making decisions about optimal drugs. If we have team members that are on medications - healthy enough to deploy, but on medications - the pharmacists can organise getting additional medications for deployment so someone can have their own cache of their medication that they could keep in their deployment bag, and that is managed by the pharmacist. The pharmacists also manage a small supply of travel medicines. When we're travelling with the team, we have medications, so we can support if someone gets ill or injured during transit. A lot of times it's just simple stuff like making sure we've got a good stash of motion sickness medicine (e.g., when you're sitting in the back of cargo plane for a while). **The pharmacists are very important in that. They also participate in all of our disaster drills and training; basically, simulating their role that they would have in the field."** *Robert replies.*

## Hurricane Katrina Experience

*Dr. Dunne jumps back in and says,* "I neglected to mention a couple of things." **There's often a partially intact framework that still exists in a community even after a disaster, so maybe there's still some local pharmacies that are open and supportive**. Our DMAT pharmacist often serves as a liaison to that. Again, back to the example of Hurricane Katrina, there were some pharmacies that were still open and had inventory, so I was able to write a prescription and my pharmacist was able to liaison with the local pharmacist and get prescriptions filled so we weren't necessarily just using our drug cache and we were helping patients maybe get a little bigger supply than we could provide for them by working with the local pharmacists. There's a number of roles in the response phase. If we get into the recovery side, part of that is the assessment of the community as we're transitioning back to normal operations. One of the things that we see - and I'm sure you guys see this all the time - is that recovery of one part of the community could take much longer than another part. **Our pharmacists on our team serve as part of the assessment to determine if a community is ready for us to pull some of the support back**. They can look at inventory. They can work with suppliers and pharmacists to help them get back to normal. At the same time, they can also help on the team side to make sure that all of our drugs and administration stuff - needles, syringes, bottles for filling prescriptions and all those things are up to date. They also compile the data. Even before we were using electronic records, we would get a report from our pharmacists at the end of every deployment about every medication used and about every prescription filled so that we had some sense of what our scope of work and impact was".

## Specific Pharmacists' Roles

"What are your thoughts on pharmacists assisting in first response?" *I ask.* "I guess it all depends on how you define first response. We often refer to first response as the non-medication stuff, in which case they wouldn't have a big role, they would be in the next wave. But, if we're looking at first response as a more comprehensive first response like a rescue type response where we would be providing medications, particularly acute care medications in the field, then I'd say that they are very very important". *Robert adamantly suggests.*

"What about first aid and wound care?" *I continue asking about previously described pharmacists' roles found in literature.* "First aid, probably less important as there are plenty of others that are capable of that. Wound care is a bit more complex. We ended up doing a lot of recurrent wound care after certain disasters where there was not much local infrastructure. Maybe I'd see a patient four or five times over the course of the week, in which case I'm doing debridement and I'm using various topicals, in which case the pharmacist would be very important to that, particularly to compound solutions that we might use for taking care of wounds". *Robert explains thinking out loud.*

"Triaging and screening in evacuation centres or attending to the walking wounded?" *I ask, not sure if I'm going to like the answer.* "That's an interesting point. We do have all of our pharmacists trained to do that. Do you need to be a pharmacist to do triaging? No, but when we're in the early phase of the disaster, anyone who might not have an intense role right then is all trained to do that. I think that's important. The screening, once you get past triage the screening, particularly medication re-conciliation. That's a huge part of our screening in disasters - sorting out what medications people are on. **The pharmacists are some of the most valuable people in that.**" *Dr. Dunne responds.*

"Prescribing continuing chronic disease medications". *I say and pause.* "Absolutely, our pharmacists were vital in especially knowing what an appropriate substitution might be. Generally, our disaster drug caches will have one medication out of each class of common drugs, well a good stock of it: one angiotensin converting enzyme inhibitor or one selective beta blocker and things like that. It might not be what the patient was on, but the appropriate dose, therapeutic substitution is really important". *Robert passionately says.*

"What about prescribing and administering vaccinations?" *I question, wondering if perhaps these are two separate questions. Robert replies,* "Prescribing vaccinations, that's a key pharmacist role and something that we have our pharmacists do. The pharmacists can give intramuscular injections and administer vaccinations and do blood pressure testing. That's important for us because it's a huge multiplier of resources".

"Developing drug algorithms and guidelines to streamline patient di-agnosis and treatment options". *I continue down this line of inquiry, getting excited about all the different roles these DMAT pharmacists have.* "That, again, is a very important role. We have a couple of committees that work on that. I would put that as a high importance as well". *Robert exclaims.*

"Assisting in decision making on health issues and disaster health management". *I follow and Robert says,* "Yes, that is important as well. We rely on our pharmacists for a lot, particularly the most ill people; a lot of our decision support, I guess, is what we call that".

"Communication advocate between different health care professions". *I ask.* "I think that's a great role for pharmacists every day in emergency and critical care, but definitely in the disaster situation because they often have a good sense of that, and **most pharmacists are experienced enough that they can bridge the primary care specialty and emergency care world**". *Dr. Dunne replies.*

"Educating the public on health risks in disasters and identifying those most vulnerable". *I say, reading the last role off the list.* "Educating the public, maybe not as much, that's hard to do. But, identifying the most vulnerable - I think that's a really key role for pharmacists. **They also often have a very good sense of vulnerable populations just because of their medication needs.** That's a big part of how you can tell something about vulnerable populations. We use prescription data and what medications people are on, people who have high doses of insulin, brittle diabetes. We really rely on our pharmacists to identify those people". *Robert ponders.*

"Did you want to elaborate on any of these roles?" *I offer.* "I think I did that as we went along. I mean I guess **I'd just elaborate overall in the sense that, for us physicians, pharmacists are really important, and I think all of us often revolve around the pharmacist on our deployments because our patients have so many medication needs.** Again, more vulnerable people are typically the sicker, the people on more medications, and they're disproportionately affected during disasters. We see that a lot. I think the pharmacist is really helpful to us. Just day-to-day, honestly, I think a lot of us that work in the larger emergency departments that are on these teams - most of us have an emergency department pharmacist there all or most of the time, **so we're pretty reliant on pharmacists and are big supporters of pharmacists in emergencies**". *Dr. Dunne concludes.*

## Pharmacists' Roles in Preparedness and Planning

*Robert pauses and I get the impression he has more to say, so I wait and he continues,* "I think number one; is understanding some of the medical needs of the community, particularly in a community that might be prone to some natural disasters, but any community - to discuss with their individual customers about what they should have on hand, talking a little bit about the importance of some of the over-the-counter medications to have on hand and things that everybody should have. But also, a big part of that mitigation is advocating for adequate supply. **I think one of the things that we see is that sometimes, something that might not be as bad a disaster becomes a disaster because there are not adequate supplies of medication, because many places operate in this just in-time inventory fashion.** A given pharmacy at a hospital, or a community pharmacy may only have a week of medications on hand for a lot of common things that get delivered. Then you have something - even a technological disaster like a big power outage or something and/or a communications problem or a flood that's not that bad, but then you can't deliver things that are needed. I think the pharmacist's role in advocating for a realistic supply of medications. Also, one of the things we try to educate the public about is for the public to keep a supply of medication, because if you've got all your medications at home for a couple of weeks and you always have a couple of weeks of buffer, that emergency or disaster event is going to affect you or your family much less because you're not running out of your medications and your blood sugar is under control or whatever". *Robert continues to describe,* "So, **pharmacists have a big role in advocating for things like insurance reform so we can make sure patients get their medications at the appropriate time.** One of the things we see a lot of in our insurance industry, is they will only pay for a certain supply of medication and won't refill the prescription until it's within two days off being empty. That doesn't really help someone be prepared if you live in a hurricane or earthquake prone region. That's a big advocacy role for pharmacists because they often understand that better than anyone else".

## Pharmacists' Roles in Response

"What about in terms of response phase?" *I wonder out loud.* "The response phase, I think it depends on the pharmacist's job. A hospital pharmacist should be carefully monitoring the inventory during a response so that they can clearly ask for help. One of the things we see a lot worldwide is that, often healthcare institutions won't ask for help until they've just about used up all their resources, whereas if they'd asked three days ago, they would have seamless resupply. Things take a little longer in disasters. We can get resources to people, but it takes time. Having that pharmacist with some knowledge - even if they're not a disaster responder and they were that hospital's pharmacist, understanding how resupply works, how you can get help during disasters and when is really a good time to ask for that, and understanding your normal rates of use. That's one of the things.

Whereas, for community pharmacists it is understanding how the disaster system works so that they can communicate what resources they might have still available to some kind of command structure. **I've seen that there are pharmacies who are often very well stocked and supplied but didn't really have the communications plan to let disaster officials know that they still had a good supply of stuff and could provide prescriptions and over-the-counter medications to the community because of lack of communication.**" *Robert responds and takes up again.* "Then, for a pharmacist who has chosen to get involved as a disaster responder - to really be able to provide that role of helping to figure out what the patient's most pressing medical needs are, helping to prioritise what pharmacy needs we might have, and then helping to get medications to patients. Sometimes even just doing outreach, maybe a patient is not currently needing any medical evaluation from the physician, nurse, nurse practitioner side, but needs some of their medications refilled in the next few days to prevent them from decompensating, to do some outreach, get out into the community and get medications to people that are affected by the disaster. We had our pharmacist going out to various shelters just to do some of that; not people that presented for care, but just to the shelter to say what have you got? Do you have enough medications to get through the next few days? What if we evacuate you 500 miles? What are you going to do? That was really helpful". *Dr. Dunne states.*

## Pharmacists' Roles in Recovery

"Lastly, what about pharmacists' roles in the recovery phase?" *I question.* "In the recovery phase, **one is to really learn from experience, to write down their experiences, share them and complete after-action reports, so they and the industry can actually learn something**. This is another thing. Sometimes we never seem to learn anything from some of these events that we go to - we just deploy with the same stuff. Even though our last after-action report said we needed a bunch of different things in our drug cache, or we ran out of something quicker at one of the hospitals that was affected by the disaster. **I'd say that's the number one thing, is tracking what really happened and looking at and writing a decent common sense after-action report and, at the same time, participating in the planning for future responses**. Sometimes it's a little dull but getting your pharmacist to stick with whatever routine planning is going to go on in the future, I think, is really important". *Robert replies with a sigh.*

## Barriers to Pharmacists' Roles

"What do you see as any potential barriers to implementing these types of roles?" *I ask nervously.* "I think one of the key obstacles is the - I don't know the best way to say it, but the lack of understanding of people in various administrative or non-medical positions about why the pharmacist is important. When you're talking to someone's hospital administrator about why you want the pharmacist to go to the disaster committee meetings, why you want the pharmacist to be available to go to training and drills and things like that, sometimes that's a tough thing for them to understand. I think getting the word out so that administrators understand the importance of pharmacists in disasters and are willing to support that pharmacist to participate in the process, because depending on your community, you might not have a disaster for a long time, so a lot of other things become important. Even if you have a pharmacist that wants to participate, their boss, if you will, might not let them participate in a meaningful fashion. I'd say that's one thing.

But I'd also say even keeping people that are interested, keeping them interested and keeping them excited is a challenge. **I think the best way to deal with that is to do regular, fairly realistic drills so that people can actually train as they fight, if you will.** They can think about what's actually happening and be a little bit more enthusiastic or excited about it. I think doing comprehensive drills is really important, something that's showy and you make a big deal of it, you get some bells and whistles and special effects and stuff going on so that you bring your administrators and non-medical personnel down. And then lastly, I would say all those things often come down to one thing, which is money to support disaster planning and response, that sometimes the people that make budget decisions at the governmental or hospital level - if they haven't been faced recently with a disaster, they may not think that it's that important". *Dr. Dunne concludes awkwardly laughing on his last point.*

## Summing Up

"The final question I have is, what suggestions do you have for an alternative or better implementation of pharmacists into disaster health management?" *I ask.* "**Number one, I think it should be a core part of the pharmacy curriculum in pharmacy school. Number two, there needs to be engagement of community pharmacists because I would say a lot of the supply and a lot of what patients perceive is their pharmacist is the apothecary on the corner. They need to get engaged in disaster planning**". *Robert replies.* "These are some great suggestions. Thank you very much for taking the time for this interview". *I conclude.*

# 12 Evidence from the Field: Pharmacy Theme

## Introduction

The third theme we will review together is the overarching theme of 'pharmacy'. This theme encompasses the specific purpose of pharmacy during emergencies including the current context of pharmacists' roles during disaster and emergency deployments. We will also cover in this chapter the benefits of pharmacists working in emergencies and why they should be better included and integrated. While some of the content in this chapter may seem a little repetitive to our earlier discussions, they do present a different lens as these are the words of others working in the field with extensive disaster and emergency expertise. So, let's quickly revisit these important topics.

What are the core responsibilities of pharmacists in disasters and emergencies? With all the responses of the interviewees, the primary objective of pharmacists working and responding to emergencies can be summarised as – ensuring continuity of care. But what does ensuring continuity of care mean? Ensuring continuity of care covers many facets of a pharmacist's skillset and services, as pharmacists adapt their roles to meet the needs of their community. This could include logistics, vaccinations, medication reconciliation, being open and accessible, providing emergency supplies, educating and counselling patients, providing behavioural first aid (also known as psychological first aid in disaster and emergency management), providing chronic disease management, and participating in risk mitigation strategies. Just to name a few. This is not an exhaustive list of what continuity of care entails, as it is dependent on the impact of the emergency, available healthcare resources, and the community needs. However, pharmacists are trained and qualified in a vast array of skills that are essential in helping manage people in the primary care setting and avoiding exacerbations requiring tertiary and emergency care. They routinely adapt their roles, knowledge, and skills to meet the need and care requirement in front of them. Pharmacists assist their patients and community in ensuring continuity of care by keeping the pharmacy operational where possible.

DOI: 10.4324/b23292-15

We as pharmacists struggle with the challenge of quantifying or describing what we mean by continuity of care, as to us it really means – meeting the needs of people. Which is a hard concept to then put down on paper. So, let's look at some of these roles that people have talked about in terms of continuity of care in a bit more detail. But with the caveat that this is by no means an exhaustive list.

## Chronic Condition Management

Disaster-affected individuals with chronic conditions or injuries that do not require a acute medical attention are sometimes referred to as the 'walking wounded' in triage protocols. While these individuals are a lower priority on the triaging scale of emergency management, they can quickly develop acute complications if not adequately managed in a timely manner. This can result in the consumption of more of the limited healthcare resources during an emergency. Many of these 'walking wounded' can be prevented from escalating up the triage scale by ensuring continuity of medication management. By engaging pharmacists in this role, it could free up other healthcare professionals' time (e.g., physicians and nurses) to focus their attention on treating the higher acuity disaster emergencies. This is illustrated in the comments by a disaster pharmacist and a hospital ED pharmacist.

> *So, the biggest concern is making sure that chronic care needs are taken care of, because what we kind of typically see is that if chronic care needs aren't taken care of, then patients actually decompensate pretty quickly within about three to five days. We start to see blood pressure, diabetes and those kinds of things become such an issue that patients may have to go to a hospital or urgent care setting.* [I15][1]

> *In the bushfire events, it was not so much the bushfire victims [disaster-affected individuals] coming in, but rather everybody else that was left in the department while people were being attended for bushfire injuries. So, just your normal old lady with the fractured hip that was getting a little less care in the department. [Pharmacists were vital] just to ensure they had their medications appropriately charted and were receiving their pack of medications appropriately, because they weren't being given the same amount of time and attention that they may have previously, when there wasn't an event going on.* [A4][1]

## Medication Reconciliation

Medication reconciliation was considered by interviewees to be an important role for pharmacists in responding to disasters and emergencies.

Pharmacists have the expertise and time in an emergency to assist people in determining what medications they are taking, and identifying which ones are critical for them to obtain supply of immediately. It is essential to know what medications a patient is taking when they are evacuated in a disaster and are displaced from their records. This is highlighted in comment from a disaster pharmacist.

> *Hurricane Katrina we had millions of people displaced from their medications. Their pharmacies were gone, and these people were walking in and hadn't had their blood pressure medicine, their heart medicine, their diabetes medicine, for weeks. They had no idea what they were taking, and all the records were destroyed. They were gone. My pharmacists sat down with those people one at a time and talked their way through all their medications and did their best to reconstruct what they were taking and get them stabilised. [19]*[1]

## Deployment Ready

Part of the responsibility for continuity of care is in the logistics of maintaining the pharmaceutical drug cache for deployment into disaster zones. A 'drug cache' is essentially the inventory of medicines and strategic storage for rapid deployment that are ready to be moved and used immediately in disaster-affected regions. Due to the unpredictability of disasters, these drug caches need to be kept up-to-date constantly, rotating out any expired stock, and updating the kits to contain the drugs that are most likely going to be needed in the right strengths and quantities.

This role can also be translated to pharmacists working in hospitals and community settings, with the need to ensure adequate quantities of medicines are kept in stock to survive a potential impact on the supply chain. This has become challenging in recent years with the move to 'just-in-time' inventory and daily ordering to restock, reducing the product sitting on the shelf and costs tied up in slow-moving inventory. The problem with this is what happens when a disaster impacts your community, and you need to meet the increased medication needs of people and are not able to obtain restock of your supplies for days or weeks?

Additionally, pharmacists working with disaster teams typically have the responsibility to ensure all team members are up-to-date with their vaccinations to be able to be deployed at a moment's notice. These points are raised by a disaster team pharmacist and a Canadian military pharmacist.

> *I believe we have a big role because as pharmacists we are responsible to make sure the kits [pharmaceutical drug cache] are ready to be deployed on a very short notice and we are responsible to maintain all*

*the kits and there is no expired medications in the kit and because once
we know we have to deploy, we have no time to order medications. We
have to keep up-to-date and keep the kit up-to-date all the time. So, we
have a big role in the preparedness and also ... we can give our advice as
to what is kept in the kit. [I1]*[1]

*So, prevention obviously with all the vaccinations etc ... we actually
have our people quite heavily vaccinated because we never know what
environment we're going to put them into. So, we have a whole bunch of
vaccines that are mandatory for all our members so that they can be
ready to deploy. Then we have a list of other vaccinations, Yellow Fever
etc., that we might have to administer to our members in preparation
for them going into different scenarios, so they're not mandatory ones,
they're on top of you know, Japanese encephalitis or whatever have
you. [A6]*[1]

## Education

Another key aspect of ensuring continuity of care is in education.
This includes disaster-affected individuals but also the broader public.
For example, explaining how people can build their own resilience and
be prepared (e.g., do they have a reserve of their ongoing chronic disease medications, or a list of what medications they are on, evacuation
plan, etc.). And of course, pharmacists are integral for providing
information, education, and counselling on the emergency specific information and medications. This is discussed in the remarks by a US
pharmacist.

*Things like that no-one else can do. The doctors are few and far
between in disasters. Nurses aren't really good at doing those sorts of
things. Pharmacists are just perfect. Post 9/11 when the anthrax - when
we were trying to distribute medications for anthrax. They tried to have
nurses and EMTs [emergency medical technicians] and people like that
distribute the medicine, but people had lots and lots of questions and the
doctors and the nurses couldn't answer them. There were interactions,
and how to properly take it and what do I do with my kids? That was
when they brought a bunch of us [pharmacists] in from the military at
that point because they didn't have enough pharmacists to fill those
roles. [I9]*[1]

## Behavioural First Aid

Most of the participants identified behavioural first aid support (also
known as psychological first aid) as a role for pharmacists to assist
their communities in disasters and emergencies. This support involves

pharmacists looking out for the signs of when someone may be experiencing a mental health crisis and referring them onto the appropriate professional support. Pharmacists see a lot of disaster-affected individuals as people seek out pharmacies as safe havens following an emergency. They come for information, healthcare, and support. So, while pharmacists are thrust into this role during times of emergencies, we need to ensure they have the adequate support to fully be prepared to step into it. This can be challenging as pharmacists are people in that community too and often are dealing with personal impacts while professionally assisting others to manage theirs. This is highlighted in a comment by an emergency physician.

> *Well I had referred to disaster behavioural health. I think it's worthwhile for all healthcare providers really, but pharmacists in particular to be trained in disaster behavioural health, because I think we have a really important role in potentially mitigating aftereffects for disaster survivors, just in knowing how to counsel them, how to approach them, how to let them just talk about the experience that they've had. So, I think that's something that we haven't focused on and that could really have a big impact with actually pretty minimal training … I've heard it's been called behavioural first aid. So, it's not being administered by a professional, it's more of an awareness level of these are the kinds of things that you can expect, these are the kind of things that you can say to be helpful, these are the kind of things you don't say and some of the actions that you can take to be helpful. Just that minor level of awareness has made me personally more comfortable in my role as I think I'm better able to take care of patients who have been survivors of not just disasters, but other kinds of outrageous events as well. [I15]*[1]

## Context of Pharmacists' Current Roles in Disasters

It has often been mentioned that pharmacists are not utilised in disasters to their full potential, and this was again a theme. So, let's review the current context of pharmacists' roles in disasters and emergencies. While it is acknowledged that pharmacists bring a unique skillset of both logistics and clinical skills into the mix when responding to a disaster, currently in terms of emergency management there is an underutilisation of the clinical abilities and expertise of a pharmacist. The counter argument is sometimes made that when a pharmacist is included within a disaster health team, there is usually only one of them and they are needed to essentially run a pharmacy as a one-person show – doing the work of several pharmacy personnel (pharmacists, dispensary technicians, assistants, supply management personnel, and logisticians). This becomes a challenge or hurdle for pharmacists, as it is difficult to expand

and utilise all of your skills to respond to an emergency when juggling so many tasks at once without the normal assistance available. This challenge is suggested by this disaster pharmacist.

> *In country, the job is basically to do all of the roles of the pharmacy technician and pharmacist in the field hospital. So, we've got to make sure about medication security, medical supply, impress [ward stock] supply, clinical checks of all of the patients, liaising on short stock to get resupply, etc ... Everyone was saying I don't want to go on a deployment as a team of one, because the pharmacist was up at 6 and working till 10 to try and get everything done, because they were so busy in the hospital, restocking and they were involved in so many different things with the clinical work and just stock control ... So, I think that's the limiting factor, we haven't actually been able to prove that we [pharmacists] are overworked. Yeah, I know it anecdotally, but we haven't actually collected that data. [A3]*[1]

With the limited presence of pharmacists in disaster teams, there is a push by some for pharmacists to keep their focus and time on logistics which is the primary reason they are often deployed. It then becomes a tug-of-war between 'the could' versus 'the should' for pharmacists' roles in disasters. Just because a pharmacist can help in a particular way, does not automatically translate to it being in the best interest for the response team or the community. The health resources available and the health needs of the community need to be considered. For example, in a hospital practice setting, there would probably be access to multiple physicians for pharmacists to work collaboratively. However, in a cut-off community the pharmacist may not have access to other healthcare professionals and may need to perform certain roles to ensure continuity of care. So, we shouldn't be neglecting specific roles and tasks that are needed by our community during a disaster or emergency.

## Benefits of Further Inclusion of Pharmacists in Emergencies

It is well known that pharmacists as healthcare team members adds to patient safety and optimises the outcomes for patients. This is also true when it comes to disaster and emergencies, by integrating pharmacists into disaster PPRR activities, we are increasing the overall health resiliency of our healthcare system and increasing the healthcare resources that are available. Especially, considering pharmacists' roles in disasters and emergencies are not new skills but rather an adaption of their existing expertise, knowledge, and skills applied in a specific situation. This is discussed in the remarks of an US emergency physician.

*In terms of response, as I said, at [Hurricne] Katrina, particularly - having a really excellent pharmacist there was - it was just irreplaceable. We could not have functioned without the pharmacist. They were able to keep straight all the inventory, help me with substitution if I needed that, get stuff for me, pretty much the same as I would if I were working at home in a large academic hospital emergency department ... I really think pharmacists are a tremendous asset to any disaster response and actually for my everyday job as well. [110]*[1]

## Chapter Reference

1 Watson KE. The roles of pharmacists in disaster health management in natural and anthropogenic disasters. [Thesis]. QUT ePrints: Queensland University of Technology; 2019 Available from: https://eprints.qut.edu.au/130757/

# 13 Story from the Field: An Interview with Amanda Sanburg

## Introduction

Let's hear from another of the incredible people that I have met that have helped shape my perspective in this field that makes up our 'Stories from the Field'. Amanda Sanburg is an Australian pharmacist that has worked on the frontline as a disaster pharmacist in many emergencies over the years. Amanda brings us a unique perspective of local response compared to that of a medical team being deployed to a region and highlights the communication challenges in emergency response. Just a reminder that these interviews were conducted before the COVID-19 pandemic was on the horizon and these participants have provided their consent to be named along with their interview in this book.

> *I begin the interview by asking the first question* "I wanted to ask what professional perspective you are coming from". "I'm a pharmacist". *Amanda replies.*

## Amanda's Experience in Disasters

"What is your experience in dealing with unpredictable events or disasters as a pharmacist?" *I query.* "Well as I mentioned in the email, my most significant experience I suppose, was following Cyclone Pam, in Vanuatu in 2015. I had been working in Vanuatu for five years full time as Principal Pharmacist for the Ministry of Health, over two terms of employment ending in 2014 ... Cyclone Pam hit in April 2015 ... But when I realised the extent of the damage and it really was quite significant, I offered to go over and assist, which I did at my own cost. I stayed for two weeks helping them in the aftermath of Cyclone Pam. When I was working in Vanuatu, I had actually been in a category four cyclone, so I suppose I had some degree of disaster experience then. But yes, a category five cyclone was probably the biggest disaster that I have been involved in". *Amanda recalls.*

DOI: 10.4324/b23292-16

## Cyclone Pam Experience

"What kind of roles were required of you during Cyclone Pam?" *I counter.* "Well, I went back to support the principal pharmacist. Most of my work was involved with looking at donations and trying to deflect a lot of donations that were totally inappropriate. That was my main focus I suppose. I was also there to be hands on. I was working in the hospital pharmacy as many of the staff had their houses blown away, or they couldn't get to work because bridges had been washed away, or they couldn't get through on a bus or vehicle to get to work. It was easier having been there previously and I knew the pharmacy set up and staff". *Amanda states and pauses as she collects her thoughts before continuing.* "There was something like 20 to 25 different foreign medical teams in country at the time. Part of my role was assisting the logistics people within those different teams, to tell them what stock we had where and what they needed and didn't need and how to get stuff from point A to point B. A bit of a logistics role but having knowledge of what was on the country's essential medicines list is imperative. **I was making sure that clinics didn't receive medicines that were beyond the capacity and training of the local staff (health workers and nurses mainly) to use.** Some donors came in with their own doctors and pharmacists and had their own self-contained mini hospital, which was fine. **I was involved with meeting with them generally when they were leaving to ensure they only left behind useful medicines and equipment. It was often a case of deflecting unnecessary supplies that frequently get donated to the countries post disaster but end up being of little use. Disposal of these excess medicines and sundries can be difficult as facilities are often not available for appropriate destruction".** *Amanda reflects.*

"Was there much of a clinical role, or was it more based on the logistics and the donations?" *I probe.* "In that situation, probably not so much of a clinical role. I was involved in providing advice around water supply and sterilisation, how to sterilise water, because a lot of people had contaminated water tanks. Our team provided quite a bit of education on use of chlorine tablets and other ways they could get access to clean water. We fortunately didn't have a lot of cholera, typhoid or hepatitis A outbreaks in this cyclone as we'd had in other mini cyclones. Generally, we were pretty fortunate with Cyclone Pam, that it was really just patching people up who'd been cut by flying debris. My role was to primarily assist with re-establishing operations. Another aspect of my role was in the area of advocating for healthy food donations and making sure they were appropriate as we have a lot of diabetes in the islands. **It's very important that there are alternative sources of healthy food available rather than just rice and noodles. Excessive carbohydrate consumption has contributed to diabetes in these countries".** *Amanda responds and continues.*

## Communication Challenges

*Amanda lingers in her memories of working through Cyclone Pam. Then she continues,* "**What I found quite interesting, was the way in which I was side-lined, which I think stemmed from the lack of communication between the different foreign medical groups. I would have thought given that it was their job, they would be great at working with the local groups.** But I re-member speaking to one team from Hawaii, and that was all they did, they just flew into disasters and brought their own 'everything' with them. Many teams weren't particularly good at communicating with people who are on the ground. Even larger international organisations didn't know what drugs were available in their emergency packs as no one was able to find a list. For those who do it on an everyday basis, I would have thought they could have been a bit better with logistics. I just used my common sense and in the case of the emergency box contents simply opened one and made a list for circulation". *Amanda muses.*

"One day I was sitting in the offices, because it was the only place you could get internet access. I was listening to the logistician in discussion with a medico from Hawaii who was wanting some antibiotics and an otoscope and other pieces of equipment. Anyway, these supplies were supposedly in one of these emergency boxes, but all the boxes had been sent out to the remote clinics for use ... So, I interrupted and suggested he go to the central medical stores as I knew they had plenty of stock. During the cyclone, they didn't lose their stock they just lost their com-puter system and the cold room, so I knew they had stock there'. Anyway, he didn't take my advice, the next day he came in and he's asking the logistician again. I just sat there, because I thought obviously, you're not listening to me, I'll just sit here quietly and carry on doing my own thing. The logistician left the room, and the medico said to me, 'look I don't know where the central medical store is?'. I told him that I was going there in 10 minutes if he wanted to join me. In the end, we got everything that he needed, and he said to me, 'you know I've been here for a week and a half now, and you've been the most helpful person that I've come across. I'm going to go back and tell all these logisticians and other health workers how to do it - **just ask the pharmacist, they know where everything is!**' I thought well there you go, something to be said for having a pharmacist onboard. Because yes, you're right, pharmacists often get forgotten and front-line staff assume there's always going to be someone who knows what they need and where to obtain it from. No one had actually thought to utilise any of the supplies that we had in country; they were just trying to utilise supplies that were brought in from outside of the country. We had plenty of our own and no one had asked. I appreciate arriving teams cannot expect supplies to be available at points of disaster but communication, once there, could have alleviated unnecessary stock movements. Sorry for the long story to answer your

question, but I think it illustrates some of the simple yet complex challenges we face". *Amanda relays and pauses for a sip of water.*

## Pharmacists Place in Disasters

"Wow, that's so interesting. I would have thought the communication
would be the first step. So, then what is your general opinion of the role
of pharmacists in disaster health management?" *I ask.* "**I definitely think
there's a role for pharmacists in disaster health. I think logistics is a big part
of it, but it goes beyond that and knowing what's likely to be needed where
and when.** Another health worker came and wanted 200 antibiotic tablets,
and I said 'where are you stationed?', and he mentioned a small community, and as I'd been there before I knew it had a small population. I
questioned him about whether they were treating everybody in that whole
town or village, explaining that they would drain our stocks if he took
200 tablets. I told them to work out how many courses they had out there
first. He radioed back to his team, and they said, 'oh yeah, we really only
need 50'. When pharmacists ask those questions, it saves a lot of wastage.
Some logisticians wouldn't think to question an order, but **a pharmacist
would as they understand the use, dosages, and implications of medications**". *Amanda recounts.*

## Pharmacists' Roles in Emergencies – Logistics or Clinical or Both?

"Do you see there being a difference between the logistics and clinical
roles that pharmacists could provide in a disaster?" *I query.* "Well yes,
there's definitely a difference. Pharmacists can potentially provide both
roles, they have experience with distribution and know the use of drugs.
**That's the advantage that a pharmacist brings to a logistics role – knowing
what alternatives can be used if you don't have something.** For instance, if
you run out of penicillin, in many cases Cotrimoxazole can be used as an
alternative, but a logistician doesn't know these things. They just place an
additional, potentially expensive air freighted order to get some penicillin.
**You're still using your clinical skills; it may not be what people think of as
the clinical role that a pharmacist has in this day-and-age but it's still using
that skillset.** I strongly advocate for pharmacists to be put into roles as
managers in charge of central medical stores. Often in the developing
countries, they put logisticians in these roles, but they have no training
around what the drugs are for, and they don't bring those extra skills and
knowledge to the table - sure they might have more experience in getting
supplies from point A to point B, but they don't understand about the
drugs. Also, pharmacists are going to be more respected when you approach a doctor. **Doctors and nurses appreciate your knowledge of drugs
and are going to listen to your recommendations of alternatives.** This may

not be the case with logisticians. **Additional roles for pharmacists in this setting could be to continue to prescribe chronic disease medicines to free the physicians up to see more difficult patients.** Pharmacists can undertake many other roles and assist with guideline-led prescribing, it just depends on the needs of the community that has been impacted". *Amanda says.* "So really the clinical and logistics go hand in hand?" *I follow, wanting to clarify.* "Yes, they do, I don't think you can really separate them. I know they do have and need logisticians, but I don't think that they are as effective as pharmacists in that role around medicines distribution". *Amanda responds.*

## Training and Skills

"What training / skill did you find helpful in your roles?" *I ask.* "Having worked for many years in the Pacific, I knew pharmacy departments distribute not just medicines but also medical supplies and equipment. I learnt a lot about different types of catheters, cannulas, and medical equipment whilst teaching pharmacy in the Solomon Islands. **I think it would be beneficial for pharmacists responding to disaster events to learn more about medical supplies and equipment.** Pharmacy in the developed world tends to only manage medicines whereas in countries like Africa, India or the Pacific Islands, they will expect you to know about medical equipment and supplies like catheters, cannulas and sutures as well". *Amanda responds, and I think yeah she's right, I was never trained in managing medical equipment or as I've read in other research, pharmacy often also look after blood and laboratory supplies and tasks.*

*Amanda continues,* "it's also **understanding about things like essential medicines list**[1] **and standard treatment guidelines,** which are basically the lists of medicines that each of these countries have approved for use in country and guidelines for their use. It is imperative for disaster teams and visiting health teams in non-disaster times to be familiar with these local documents and abide by them where possible. Many visiting health teams come into country and they bring in non-essential drug list medicines that often get left behind once the teams leave. If these foreign teams could use the essential drug list (EDL) medicines that we have in country, it would be that much more helpful for the local staff. Local staff will see the use of their medicines, rather than medicines that others bring in and they will learn their application. Using non-EDL medicines simply increases the dependence on the external team".

"Donation guidelines[2] are another important document to be familiar with. So many people believe that you want donations of medicines and equipment. In reality, they are not necessarily in the best interest of countries in any situation except possibly when the stores have all been completely wiped out. In Cyclone Pam, most of the drugs that were brought in, were brought in by each team and none of the medicines that we had in stock were used. It was quite an unusual situation because people just completely forgot about the local resources and brought in their own supplies, at no doubt great expense, when there were adequate supplies on their doorstep to be used, if they needed it". *Amanda passionately explains.*

## Pharmacists' Role in Managing Donated Medicines

*I begin preparing to ask my next question but realise that Amanda is collecting her thoughts and has more to say, so I stay silent. Amanda resumes,* "Also, **I think a big role for pharmacists is in deflecting unnecessary donations. The donations can just be ridiculous. I calculated that I must have stopped at least two million US dollars' worth of donations from coming to Vanuatu after that cyclone.** There were donations that would never have been of any use and then difficult to appropriately dispose of. There were things like a higher strength of nifedipine and the wrong form of gentamicin compared to our EDL, or stocks that were going to expire in the next three months. Things like 50,000 jars of face cream, I'm thinking – 'why do we need 50,000 jars of face cream post cyclone?' It was just crazy, the stuff that was being sent. The donors were going to send us all this short-dated stock and excess stock that they'd collected from various companies and write it off against their tax as a donation. **I went through and worked out that at best we would have been able to use 7–8% of the supplies that they'd offered us.** These supplies were already packed up and ready to go, but I intervened and stopped it. I wasn't very popular with the people who'd packed it all up! But, that's a very important role for pharmacists, because not everybody has the time in a disaster to actually look at this level of detail. Other countries think we want them to send drugs, that we need drugs, but nobody asks the staff on the ground. The number of donations that get sent, that are totally inappropriate or not necessary, is ridiculous!" *Amanda adamantly describes.*

"How did you deflect them from coming?" *I wonder aloud.* "Well, because I'd worked in the central medical stores, I was asked to review a list of donated medicines that the stores team had said yes to initially. After going through the list, I came back to the team and discussed with them that while the names of the drugs were used in country, the dosage form or strength was not and could potentially cause medical errors. For example, nifedipine 90 mg sustained release was being sent but we only use the 20 mg tablets or gentamicin minibags (a delivery vessel not available in Vanuatu) 360 mg and we only kept 80 mg in 2mLs ampoules. **Those differences could result in dispensing/administration errors in these countries because people aren't familiar with different strengths and different forms of products. It just helps to have someone a bit more pedantic or detailed-oriented I suppose and prepared to check every detail which is what pharmacists do every day".** *Amanda explains, and I imagine that* *conversation happening with her and the medical stores team.* "We had another group came to us, wanting to give donations of particular equipment. I actually sat down with the local advisor to midwifery and one of the central medical stores staff. We went through and requested only pieces of equipment that we really needed. That is where donations can be helpful, when the donating organisation is willing to meet the stated needs of the disaster-affected community and not the assumed needs. It is imperative to speak to the local staff of their actual needs". *Amanda concludes.*

## Pharmacists' Important Role in Disaster Planning

"Where do you believe pharmacists could have a role in the four phases - prevention, preparedness, response and recovery of a disaster?" *I question.* "All of them really. One of the issues that we came across was when the airport was upgraded and the staff were trained, they realised that they have no disaster management plan in place, in case of a plane crash. They came to us and said we need this list of drugs. I asked them why they needed these drugs, because there were things like morphine and other sedatives on their list. They explained that was what they were supposed to have in the event of a disaster. I asked them for their disaster action plan, and what staffing was available to ad-minister these emergency drugs? Who's going to be the person attending to this? They said they'd just ring the hospital, and someone will have to come. I gave a confused look and explained that the hospital would also need a plan in that case and probably would want to bring their own drugs. No-one had actually thought through the process, they just thought if they had the drugs sitting there, they'd be fine. More wor-ryingly, the hospital did not have any disaster action plans either, **so it all became a huge task that pharmacy essentially directed, because there was nobody else thinking about planning and preparing for this type of potential disaster**". *Amanda responds.*

## Pharmacists' Roles in Disaster Preparedness

"What roles do you think pharmacists could undertake in specifically preparing the community for a disaster or a natural hazard?" *I question.* "I suppose safety issues and basic first aid, assisting in education about basic first aid and having a small first aid kit at home. Regarding food, in the olden days in the islands they used to store some of their food in the ground, specifically for disasters like cyclones and tsunamis. When the disaster struck, they could go and dig up the buried dried bread-fruit, to have some source of food in the days following that cyclone. Educating communities about water sterilisation in the event of con-tamination is also an important area of preparedness. I think there's a big role for basic first aid training, it doesn't necessarily have to be a pharmacist who does that, but it doesn't hurt for them to be involved. Pharmacists need to be involved in compilation of drug kits as they are familiar with what the country stocks, prices, availability etc. I think pharmacy has a big role to play in all of these areas, definitely in preparedness". *Amanda replies.*

## Pharmacists' Roles in Emergency Response

"What about in regard to the response phase?" *I continue the line of inquiry.* "I think the most important thing is getting the right drugs that are needed to the places where they need to be in the appropriate quantities, and managing overzealous donors, so that they're adhering to the EDL and standard treatment guidelines". *Amanda explains.*

## Pharmacists' Roles in Disaster Recovery

"What about in terms of recovery and learning from previous disasters to inform future ones?" *I ask.* "We had a debrief after the disaster about some of the issues that came up and some of the things that we needed to improve before the next cyclone. Cyclones are a common occurrence in the Pacific but fortunately lower than Category five although you never know until it hits how damaging it will be ... As mentioned earlier, reviewing of disaster plans and ensuring the medical stores provide copies of the EDL, equipment lists etc. will all help in future events. There are lots of areas for pharmacist to be involved in. I think in all those four areas, there was a role we played". *Amanda responds.*

## Barriers to Pharmacists' Roles in Emergencies

"What do you see as the barriers to implementing these types of roles?" *I question, hoping for some barriers that might be easy to address.* "**Nobody thinks to take a pharmacist along**. I was very impressed that the Australian team came and brought their own pharmacist. I went and had a chat to him wondering what his experiences were. He was a nice guy and keen but really, he was very much kept dispensing, that was his job, he'd been brought along to be the dispenser and that was it. He wasn't involved with any of the other activities, I don't think he ever got outside of their hospital tent. When I went to see him, he was about to have some lunch and he brings out a packet of dried food and boiled the water. He explained he was a bit sick of dried food after a week and a half, and I suggested he visit a coffee shop downtown and support the local economy. He said, 'you're kidding me, they've actually got shops functioning?' He was just cocooned inside this tent because he was just dispensing the whole time. I thought 'this is hardly a riveting role to be playing'. He hadn't even gone and introduced himself to the local staff". *Amanda explains and suggests,* "**I think a lot of it is uncertainty about roles and about familiarity with pharmacists' roles in disasters and the rest of the team. For pharmacists with no experience in working in developing countries, there may be concerns about overstepping your mark**". *Amanda concludes and continues,* "I think that's the advantage of me and other volunteer pharmacists going back there. There were three pharmacists who went after Cyclone Pam, me and two colleagues. We had all worked in Vanuatu, and because we'd all worked there previously, they were happy for us to come back. We had other pharmacists who had volunteered to assist as well, but the country only wanted people who'd worked with them before. I think that could be a stumbling block, because the local people want people who are familiar with their operational systems and know the staff, the people, the culture. That's a very important thing, particularly in the islands at least anyway, that people are familiar with you and feel comfortable with you. They don't have to spend all their time explaining to you how the system works, because you can just pick up and go. Generally, you know what needs to be done. They trust you to work in their best interests. I think that's where bringing in external people could be a challenge. I could also act as a conduit with the foreign teams. There were daily meetings for an hour and a half every morning in the international command offices, for about four weeks. The senior pharmacy staff should have gone to those meetings everyday but they felt intimidated by so many foreigners and left them to go about it. The staff went back to their workplaces and carried on their normal duties. **It appeared as though the teams were competing amongst themselves at times and local involvement appeared limited and at times disregarded. I am sure the whole process could have been better managed with fewer teams and better communication amongst themselves and more importantly with the local services**". *Amanda summarises.*

## Enablers for Pharmacists' Roles in Disasters

"Wow, that is a very interesting perspective, thank you for sharing it with me. How do you think we can address these barriers?" *I wonder and ask, not sure how you improve communication from organisations with different perspectives, ideas, and stakeholders.* "Well first of all governments and aid organisations have to acknowledge that pharmacists have got a role to play in disasters … I suspect it's probably just for the logistics roles at this point, but **it'll be like 'clinical pharmacy', they never thought we needed pharmacists in the hospital wards, and now we're everywhere, so it'll just take time. Hopefully it'll take less time and people will acknowledge and appreciate the value of having a pharmacist on board for all aspects of disaster work**". *Amanda considers.*

## Summing Up

"How to do it, I'm not too sure. I suppose just having people on the ground or include people who have a working knowledge of that area. I suppose it's just a case of appreciating that pharmacists do form part of the team. I think that's happening, it's happening faster in the islands than it ever did in Australia. There was much more resistance in Australia because health professions are much more protective of our assumed professional boundaries. In the Pacific Islands, they're very accepting of having pharmacists as part of the team. The problem is there just aren't enough pharmacists. They have to get enough staff to start with, before people start to appreciate that there's a role for pharmacists in that whole process. **But it's starting to happen. The local pharmacists need to stand up and be confident in their skillset and promote their capacity to be included in the team.**" *Amanda says thinking out loud.*

"Thank you so much for sharing your perspective and experience with me. It sounds like you've had a very interesting and rewarding career working in the Pacific Islands". *I compliment and make my goodbyes.*

## Chapter References

1 World Health Organization. *WHO model list of essential medicines.* 20th Edition. World Health Organization; 2017.
2 World Health Organization. *Guidelines for medicine donations revised 2010.* WHO Press, Geneva, Switzerland: World Health Organization; 2010.

# 14 Evidence from the Field: Barriers and Enablers Theme

## Introduction

The last theme we will review together is the overarching theme of 'barriers and enablers'. It's important for us to stop and consider, well if pharmacists are integral in disasters as we have discovered, why aren't they already more involved? To answer this question, we will review the external and intrinsic barriers. The external being what is outside of a pharmacist's control and intrinsic being what is within their control. We will also look at external and intrinsic enablers that could increase pharmacists' involvement and integration in emergency management. These barriers and enablers are from the viewpoint and perspective of the people interviewed and what they believe to be limiting pharmacists' roles in disasters and what factors could enable the progression of pharmacists' integration in disasters as team members.

## External Barriers

The external barriers identified by the interviewees are those which limit pharmacists' progression and are believed to be outside a pharmacist's control. The first major barrier identified by some of the interviewees is the social stigma that pharmacists just 'stick labels on boxes'. So, what could they possible contribute to this space of emergency management? This is discussed in the comments from a disaster pharmacist.

> *You think about in hospitals when doctors do the ward rounds with all the registrars and there are some consultants that say, I am not going on a ward round unless the pharmacist is there, because I need to know the pharmacy side of things. Others that just go, no, no, there's no need for a pharmacist. We'll always have those barriers because they see us as people that put labels on boxes. [A6]*[1]

The perception of others is not something that we can easily rectify. But individual pharmacists can influence their colleagues by contributing to

DOI: 10.4324/b23292-17

everyday collaborations regarding their patient's management. The biggest change to this stigma will take a collective effort and strong advocacy from our global pharmacy partners. I would suggest we need a big global media campaign that tackles the question – what does a pharmacist do? The pharmacy profession has evolved drastically over the last few decades and yet, we haven't brought the public along with us. They are often unaware of the advance scope of practice pharmacists have in many regions.

A suggested barrier that is believed to partly explain the exclusion of pharmacists in emergency management is the lack of awareness by other healthcare professionals, disaster management personnel, and administrators on what pharmacists' roles could and should be in emergencies. Pharmacists are often viewed as either an unnecessary resource or a support service and not identified as an essential member of the team. This is illustrated in the remarks from an international experienced US disaster pharmacist.

> *I can't tell you how many times I've had pharmacists be cut out of critical roles and the answer has always been come on, if we need somebody, we will call on you guys, but you don't need to be here for this. [19]*[1]

Again, this is not a simple solution that a single pharmacist can tackle. While we have influence over our individual spheres, it requires a consolidated team effort across the profession to enact real change in this area. Many of the interviewees mentioned that if there was clarity on the job description of pharmacists' roles in disasters, perhaps other healthcare professionals would be more comfortable and willing to include them in additional roles and as team members.

> *I think if medical professions that are involved in disaster management had greater awareness of what skillsets pharmacists had and what role they could play, I think that might help champion and facilitate greater involvement and maybe help us more clearly define what the role is. Rather than this ad hoc and it just happens and then you figure out what you need to do. [12]*[1]

Job security was raised as a barrier for pharmacists to leave their regular employment and go on deployment which could lead to reduced staff capacity of pharmacy personnel to run the pharmacy. Additionally, pharmacy staff can be personally affected by the disaster or not physically able to get to the pharmacy which also can reduce staff capacity. Another issue for community pharmacy owners in a disaster is the dilemma of balancing their pharmacist ethical and moral duty of care decisions with their business owner lens and financial considerations. It is known that when people are evacuated, they often leave without their medications or money. Additionally, with power outages associated with emergency events the payment systems in pharmacies could not be working. This leads to pharmacists providing medications, services, and items free of charge. However, as business owners they need to consider the financial implications of providing free medications on the business' bottom line. If a community pharmacy is already experiencing financial vulnerability, providing free medications and services to the community without subsequent compensation from the government could see the pharmacy close because of the disaster. It is a difficult choice to be made by owners of small pharmacies and it comes down to the individual pharmacist and business owner's judgement on how they choose to respond with regards to their pharmacy. This was highlighted in the interviews by two different Australian pharmacists' perspectives.

> *A lot of times we end up doing things for nothing and we don't get remunerated and it doesn't pay the bills unfortunately. If there was some sort of remuneration package associated with it, not a problem ... I know other pharmacies within our retail environment definitely wouldn't do it ... It comes down to us and what do we get paid to do this? As an ex-owner, if you don't pay the rent you go broke. So, you can do all these things and it's all good, but you need to get renumerated in a business sense. [A8]*[1]

> *We were just giving vital or urgent medicines and antibiotics and painkillers, and I was just giving it to patients, because I couldn't charge them anyway. It was ridiculous to even think ... The day after [the disaster], I didn't charge anyone for anything ... . It was just a write-off. [A12]*[1]

Community pharmacies sometimes may not be given the option to make the decision to assist in a disaster depending on their location. For convenience, many pharmacies can be found in shopping centres or malls and can therefore be bound by the opening or closing of the shopping complex in the event of a disaster.

## Intrinsic Barriers

External barriers are not the only potential obstacle we need to navigate when preparing and responding to emergencies. There are intrinsic barriers which are more within an individual pharmacist's capabilities to change and could allow them to be more involved in emergencies. One of the major factors discussed by the interviewees of this study was the individual pharmacist's confidence in their expertise and skills to respond to an emergency. This is highlighted in the following two comments from pharmacists.

*In my opinion, many pharmacists would think, someone else could be doing that. … So, I think in many of the cases the barriers would be the pharmacists themselves not feeling either competent or resourced to be able to fill most of those roles. [A4]*[1]

*All of a sudden, all that stuff I learned in pharmacy school that I rarely used in a retail environment [community pharmacy] became really necessarily and useful and I've been doing this ever since. [I9]*[1]

Additionally, it is believed that pharmacists' do not perceive themselves as a first responder or essential to emergency management with some going one step further and suggesting pharmacists' do not even see themselves as healthcare providers.

*I think part of it is they don't see themselves as healthcare providers. They see themselves as retail. [I14]*[1]

Some interviewees suggested pharmacists are currently not more involved in disasters because there is a lack of interest from the pharmacy profession, and they speculated that this may be because there is a lot of competition for their time. This is illustrated in the remarks by a disaster emergency physician.

*The biggest barrier is that there is so much demand already for issues, medical issues. Preparation for disasters is just one of many things that civic leaders, medical civic leaders have to contend with. Whether it's chronic care, access to care, care for people with disabilities. There's no limit of possibilities for an individual to volunteer for or to spend their extra time in. So, that's the biggest challenge I think is just the competition for a health care professional's time and where she or he must decide what their side project, their avocation, their extracurricular interests are going to be. That's just the challenge. [I3]*[1]

Let's not focus solely on the negatives and barriers to pharmacists' roles in emergencies and review some of the enablers to pharmacists' taking their place in emergency management.

## External Enablers

The people that were interviewed were asked to provide suggestions and recommendations on how pharmacists could be better integrated into disaster health management and disaster teams. It was noted that although there are barriers, if the collective 'we' wanted pharmacists to be more involved and included, there are always work-arounds to be explored (e.g., distributing current pharmacists' workload on deployment). This is demonstrated in the quote from a Canadian military pharmacist.

> *But at the same time, if we really wanted to have more responsibilities, we can redistribute some of the workload — like the resupply of the medical material can be done by say a nurse and then the pharmacist could do more of a bigger scope of practice. There are constraints but there are always solutions if we really want the pharmacists playing new roles. [I1]*[1]

Additionally, it was put forward that we could have pharmacists working under remote orders to backfill prescribing roles as needed (for regions that don't have prescribing pharmacists). This is highlighted in the comments by a UK emergency physician.

> *It might be something that would have to be in the event of a disaster they're allowed to do these things or if communications can be done like what we do with paramedics - we give remote orders. We just give orders over the phone. There's probably no reason in certain instances that a community pharmacy - couldn't be attached to a physician who could also, under those conditions, give them the orders that they need to deliver those medications or that care within their scope. [I12]*[1]

To improve communication and collaboration between the different healthcare professionals, it was suggested to form a healthcare coalition. These groups or coalitions should regularly review emergency preparedness, response, and recovery plans. Pharmacists should also participate in interprofessional preparedness activities like scenarios, table-top exercises (TTX), or drills. It was also discussed that pharmacists need to get actively involved in disaster management, whether volunteering with NGOs or developing their skills in mass gathering medicine (i.e., large sporting events and festivals) to prepare for disasters and emergencies. Some of the interviewees suggested there needs to be a review of insurance reform. In North America in particular, insurance companies can set restrictions on how soon patients can refill their prescriptions, meaning patients may not be able to build up personal reserves especially in high-risk disaster-prone areas or be able to get an early refill after evacuating without their medications.

There was a proposal made by the interviewees for the sharing of dispensing histories and databases in the event of a disaster or emergency. This could ensure pharmacists and healthcare professionals in the community have access to patients' medical histories and patients in a community have access to the right medications. While I acknowledge there are some challenges with proprietary information for pharmacies from a business sense, there must also be some flexibility to respond to emergency situations. Countries that have electronic health records that include patient's medication histories does make this a little easier to navigate for pharmacists.

## Intrinsic Enablers

The interviewees provided some recommendations on things pharmacists themselves can do to raise awareness for better integration of their roles in disasters and emergencies that are more within their control. Primarily they recommended that we as pharmacists need to advocate for our place in emergency management and ensure our presence is known. We can each individually begin doing this within our sphere of influence and together this can begin to make a substantial change. This is demonstrated in the comments by a UK emergency physician.

> ... *my thinking is it's really something that the pharmacists really need to step up and demonstrate their role and the importance of their role both in the development and the distribution - and logistics of distributing medications - but also being the ones that connect directly to the people in the community that are vulnerable or need the medications. [I12]*[1]

Also, due to pharmacists' daily interactions with the community, we can identify those individuals who are most vulnerable to adverse health outcomes as a result of a potential disaster or emergency. For example, as we discussed earlier in this book about the various adverse health outcomes commonly associated with specific emergency events and how medications can play a factor in increasing people's vulnerability and susceptibility. We can provide public health messaging to our patients to assist them in preparing for emergencies and educate them on having personal reserves of medications and first aid kits. This is highlighted in the comments by a US emergency physician and a US pharmacist.

> *The public health message about making sure do you have enough of your medications. Keeping a personal cache of medications available in case you can't get to the pharmacy. I think those kinds of things would be, like public service announcements and those sorts of things would be popular in terms of how they prepare the public. [I10]*[1]

Pharmacists can also provide written information sheets to assist with counselling large volumes of patients in a mass casualty or prophylaxis campaign following a disaster or emergency. In line with pharmacists' role in information and documentation, it was recommended that pharmacists take an active role in writing post-disaster after-action reports. These reports would include discussions on what worked well in the emergency response, what challenges were faced by pharmacists in their communities, and how the pharmacy response can be improved for future emergencies. This is not an exhaustive list but it's a good place to start.

While there are some barriers to pharmacists working in disasters and emergencies as listed earlier, there are also things we can do now both within our individual sphere of influence and collectively to further the integration and recognition of pharmacists' place in emergencies. I challenge each and everyone one of us reading this book to consider how you can be a part of the positive change we want to see in this space.

## Chapter Reference

1 Watson KE. *The roles of pharmacists in disaster health management in natural and anthropogenic disasters.* [Thesis]. QUT ePrints: Queensland University of Technology; 2019 Available from: https://eprints.qut.edu.au/130757/

# 15 Story from the Field – An Interview with Captain Tim Davis

## Introduction

The last person I would like to introduce you to in this book is, Captain Tim Davis. Captain Davis has worked for several years in disaster management with various roles including chief medical officer, disaster epidemiologist, as well as roles within the military. This interview has some unique insight from a physician who has worked closely with pharmacists in the field responding to emergencies and has been a champion for pharmacists being recognised in the emergency management space. The 'Stories from the Field' interviews were conducted before the COVID-19 pandemic was on the horizon and these participants have provided their consent to be named along with their interview in this book.

*I met Captain Tim Davis at the 2017 WADEM Congress held in Toronto, Canada. I was in the beginning phases of my PhD journey, and I was conducting a survey of the international delegates to begin to identify pharmacists' roles in disasters. I came up to Capt. Davis and gave the spiel about the survey and how I wanted to find out if pharmacists have a place in disasters and would he consider please filling it out and returning it to the administration table. He paused and gave me a quizzical look and* said "I'm going like what? It's like do pharmacists have a role in disasters. I'm going like oh my goodness why are you asking?* **Pharmacists are already working in disasters, so of course they have a place on the team. I rely on my pharmacists in the field as a physician It's just a strange question from my perspective."** *I paused, a little taken a back as this did not match the research I had conducted so far or my own personal experience.* "Um, if you ask people in Australia, you get a very different response, can I please interview you for the next stage of my study?" *I plead. I begin the interview with my prepared informed consent spiel and asked the typical question of what country Capt. Davis is from and what his profession is, he responded,* "The United States and I am a physician".

DOI: 10.4324/b23292-18

## Captain Davis' Experience in Disasters

"What is your experience in dealing with unpredicted events or disasters in your profession?" *I question.* "My immediate past position was the Chief Medical Officer, CMO of the US National Disaster Medical System (NDMS). Prior to that Centre for Disease Control, where I was a disaster epidemiologist. I've had various other positions in disasters, in the military and elsewhere. But those cover the last 15 years". *Tim explains and I think about the wealth of knowledge he must have from all of these positions.* "What roles were required of you during these events?" *I continue.* "Various roles over the years. I've served as a medical clinician. I've served as an epidemiologist. I've served various roles in public health, working with the various Ministries of Health after the event. Basically, looking for unmet needs where public health could help build up the infrastructure, take advantage of the situation to help raise the level of public health during the area. Also, in actual management of a disaster, moving medical resources, making decisions about what we should do, what the standard of care was, scope of practice, how to assist but not cause negative impact on the local medical community by us coming in and giving free care". *Capt. Davis states.*

"In those roles, was your scope of practice ever stretched and in what way?" *I respond, wondering if the question makes enough sense.* "It's always stretched. Many different ways. One is that just because you're capable of doing it, doesn't mean you should do it. In other words, you can helpbut if you leave the community with an inability to take care of that person or the person could not survive in that community afterwards, then you can't necessarily do everything that you possibly know how to do. Often you have to improvise with what limited resources you have, and you have to make do. **Sort of fight the war with the army you can, not the army you want**. So, there's compromises every which way. I generally find that those people who have served in the military understand this because they know how to take orders. People that have not worked in the military, physicians in particular, they're not used to taking orders from anybody, but are used to being independent decision makers without limitations. They have more of a problem in these types of events". *Tim explains.*

## Concept of 'Do No Harm' in Emergency Response

"What about in relation to a team atmosphere? say for a local disaster or something like that where you've got more in relation to healthcare resources, does it change then?" *I ask, appreciating the perspective of 'do no harm' and how it needs to be applied in a disaster situation.* "It changes a lot. So, if I'm responding inside like the United States for example that's a developed country, there's all sorts of, laws, rules, regulations but they can be suspended at times. **It's mainly about supplementing the locals and trying to assist them without again causing harm**. Because again the care we give is free and the local providers, for example in the United States is fee-for-service model or it's a private medical system. So, the local providers cannot compete with our free federal care. We can end up putting them out of business or can disrupt the patient-physician relationship that they have there. In your case, like in the pharmacy world, they can't compete with our free medications. After Hurricane Katrina, the hurricane that hit New Orleans for a good bit of time, the Governor of the State of Mississippi kicked us out after about six weeks appropriately, because we were starting to impact the commercial ventures of his pharmacists, hospitals, and physicians. Whereas, in Louisiana, they have more of a history of social care, and they would not let us leave. We ended up staying there about six months rather than just six weeks. The local physicians and pharmacies could not compete with us, they actually closed, and they moved from the rural areas to more profitable parts of the state or just frankly moved out of the state. But Hurricane Katrina was in 2005 and so when I went back to Louisiana in 2010, the same impact area, but this time it was the Deepwater Horizon oil spill disaster. I went there and the physician's office, pharmacies, and hospitals where we had been there for a long period of time were closed and had remained closed". *Tim describes.* "Wow, that's an interesting perspective I had not considered before, thank you for sharing". *I responded and was momentarily silent as I reflected on this new aspect of emergency response that I hadn't considered before.*

## Unique Challenges in Responding to the Haiti Earthquake

"Is it a common occurrence then for someone with your skillset in these types of situations to have your scope of practice stretched?" *I ask, wondering how people set boundaries while responding to crises.* "It's both ways. It's stretched rightly so and sometimes it's compressed. **There's always more you can do, but then the question is - should you do it? Should you provide care that the country cannot sustain after you leave?** Case example, there are no intensive care units in the entire country of Haiti. None at all. So how do you manage that? What do you do to help somebody and there's no place for them to get care after you leave, or you have resuscitated them but there's no place to admit them to for ongoing care? As far as stretching, doing things outside your normal scope of practice. For me, not so much in emergency medicine, we pretty much cover the gamut. We don't do chronic care, long term care. Yet we of course end up doing it with our homeless population when they come to emergency departments for their chronic care. So, for the most part it's ... sort of moving my practice to a different setting and trying to interpret complaints of the local people so that I'm actually taking care of the correct thing". *Tim responds and recalls,* "I'll give you an example. In Haiti, the term 'grinding teeth' means you have seen worms in your stool. That's what they say. They say they're grinding teeth. So, when I'm looking at the medical records, we're getting requests for dentists, and I realised what's going on as they're doing a direct translation of what the people are complaining about. Not what the term means. It would be similar to us saying catching a cold or hay fever. Our grass does not have a temperature and we certainly don't run after a temperature change. But we know what that means. Same thing in Haiti, to say worms in your stool is very, very gauche. So, the term they have adopted is grinding teeth to mean that you have worms in your stool. You have to quickly adapt to the local culture. You would think and hope the local translators would be able to understand that. But a lot of times the local translators are the intelligentsia, the educated, and they don't know the local terms any better than you do". *Tim shares.* "Did you feel that you were fully equipped to handle the challenging circumstances of these different events?" *I enquire, wondering how Capt. Davis feels about the emergencies he has been involved in.* "I was from the physical care capability. But from my position, like in Haiti, it's a commanding control position and I had a very difficult time dealing with the other physicians who wanted to do everything and ended up again creating surviving patients who there was no place that they could be taken care of. That's the part I felt inadequate about. I had people that were routinely violating international laws and didn't understand that they have a licence in that country to practice, only because of the blessing of the host government. Yet the host government places restrictions on what we can or can't do. If we go beyond that then we are practicing without a licence. It was very difficult for me to get the physicians to understand that. I'd never had to deal with that type of situation before. In past experiences I've dealt with more uniformed service type individuals, and they understood restrictions and orders and things like that. I've worked with individuals like this before, but that's working with them, not in a command situation during a disaster response". *Tim recounts.*

## Pharmacists' Place in Disasters

*Changing course I ask,* "What is your personal opinion on the role of pharmacists in disaster health management?" *hoping Tim hasn't changed his mind since we first spoke at the WADEM congress.* "**It's critical. We talked before about it. But it's actually critical. They're probably one of the key individuals we need to have.** This is from everything from interpreting local drugs, substitutes for the drugs we're used to, getting the medications, making decisions on when we're throwing a temperature log or particular drug on deciding what the priority is for the special request. Everything from soup to nuts actually. The group I just left, the National

Disaster Medical System. We had three full time pharmacists and one full time physician - the Chief Medical Officer physician". *Tim passionately explains.*

"What do you think about the pharmacists' roles in the recovery phase or would that be returning to normal business for pharmacy?" *I ask.* **"Back to normal business. It extends far beyond that. Recovery actually will go on for years.** We still have people working for recovery from Hurricane Sandy, which was the hurricane that hit New York City in 2012. So, this is what several years later, and we are still working on the recovery. So, it's getting things back up to normal to a point. But there's a lot of other issues that will occur, particularly people that are marginalised in their healthcare situation, that's both mental as well as physical healthcare. They generally deteriorate much more rapidly and because they've lost their social infrastructure, their way of doing things, their pattern, their ritual. This decline is often going to be observed by the pharmacist rather than the physician of a hospital who sees the person just in a 15- or 20-minute appointment in their office, you know once a month or once a year. So, recovery on the surface will look like business as usual. But it will be a long time until recovery has been completed for all those folks that were again were sort of on the brink of things before the event. Then of course you have those that just because the trauma of the event and things like this they deteriorate in other ways. But yeah, so business as usual and beyond". *Tim states and pauses before sharing another aside.*

## Pharmacy as Community Recovery Litmus Test

"What I do, and this might be a time to mention this. **When I go to a community after a disaster, I go to the local pharmacy. The pharmacy is generally the first institution that gets up and running.** They will know what physicians are in the area and whether they're operational or not. They'll know the patients that are in the area. **So, pharmacists are one of the key groups I find**. I will go and try to find the closest unaffected pharmacy that's operational and then start there and then work back towards the epicentre of the disaster. **Pharmacists have a huge role in taking care of their community. But I actually use them as a surveillance tool to find out how the community is recovering**. Hospitals take a little bit longer to do that. Physicians are mobile. So, they are victims as well as first receivers. Not first responders, but first receivers and caretakers. **But the pharmacist or the pharmacy is usually the first medical operation that's fully operational**. So, they have a key role to play in rebuilding the community. They're the ones that are going to know their community and how it's rebuilding. So, they're a key person to know what the needs are in the community, who's on insulin, who's getting nutritional feedings. Who is doing all of that? They'll be working in the community for sure, probably educating, helping people. Because if you aren't able to get your medications, then you will send the kids and the non-bread winner out of town and the bread winner generally stays behind to rebuild. However, if you have medical care there and it starts with the pharmacy, then the family will generally stay intact and will work on rebuilding the community". *Tim shares from his perspective of the vital place pharmacy has in the community, being a community landmark following a disaster or emergency.*

## Disaster and Emergency Health and Pharmacists' Scope of Practice

"Do you think assisting in disasters is within pharmacist current scope or practice?" *I follow up.* "Yes, again they're a critical key. They understand the logistics process. They understand and can help make decisions about prioritisation. They can make decisions about substitutions, interpretation of local drugs, local standards, alternative ways to get them. Understanding import, export licensing, narcotics law internationally and nationally" *Tim says and continues,* "**They need to be involved in the entire PPRR cycle, especially preparedness.** In preparation, the drug cache is the equipment supply and in dealing with the choice of the medications, the substitutions, the quantities, the burn rate. Pharmacists have a key role in advising on substitutions. Advising on what's critical and what's not. I'll make an aside here. We have a saying; 'you can't take Walter Reed south'. Walter Reed is our largest military medical hospital. So, you can't take the entire hospital with you, and you can't take your entire pharmacy with you or the entire hospital formulary with you. You have to be able to make decisions and substitutions and decide what is really critical and what is not critical. The pharmacist will know because of their dealings in the day-to-day with the physicians on what is really absolutely critical and what is the physician just posturing that they need/want this drug, because it's their favourite drug". *Tim responds and I am stunned with how passionately Capt. Davis advocates for pharmacists' place in disasters.*

## Mass Gathering Medicine

"I would look for ways you could prepare in just small types of disasters or pending disasters. This could be getting involved in mass gathering medicine … Get involved in those types of things. It could just be local festivals. But you go in and you prepare. Or, you have a big influx of tourists in the town for a special event and you try to go through what the demands are for your pharmacy workplace. What would the increased demands on the hospital be in casualties or impact on the emergency department. But you go through the same motions that you might need to respond to a disaster in general. **You try to do the same thing every time no matter what and you just go through the process, even though it might be relative void, you are going through the thought process preparing for an actual disaster. Plus, you can do the recruiting at the same time. And you do community education and community outreach".**

*Capt. Davis suggests.* "Thank you so much for your time and support, I am so glad that we met at the WADEM Congress". *I gush and make my goodbyes.*

# Part IV

# Practical Guide for Pharmacists Working in Disasters and Emergencies

So far, we have covered the basics of emergency management in Part I, pharmacists' place in Part II, and the evidence from the field in Part III. In the last section of this book, we are going to look at more practical aspects of pharmacists and emergency management. This includes a discussion about some of the legal and ethical considerations we have as pharmacists working in disasters and how to prepare both professionally and personally as a pharmacist. We will also work through some ways in which to teach these activities in pharmacy school with the use of a worked example. Then, finally, a conversation about the disasters and emergencies that change us.

DOI: 10.4324/b23292-19

# 16 Ethico-Legal Considerations

## Introduction

We have discussed at length the benefits of pharmacists' roles and services in disasters and outlined their place in emergency management. But with pharmacists' undertaking their full scope of practice in emergencies, there also needs to be some flexibility and consideration for the pharmacy legislation and regulations that govern the profession. Additionally, like anything in terms of healthcare, there are ethical considerations that pharmacists as healthcare professionals need to navigate. It's important we talk about this and how it impacts the emergency response from pharmacists, so we can begin advocating for change and appropriate flexibility.

The question of 'if' or 'when' pharmacists become more active in disasters is not hypothetical. Pharmacists are already performing many roles in an *ad-hoc* fashion in different capacities when a disaster impacts their community. The ethico-legal and moral issues need to be discussed and resolved to better empower and support pharmacists' roles in emergencies. So, let's review some of them. Sometimes these pharmacists are risking their lives to ensure their communities have their medications and providing pharmacy services,[1,2] and we need to ensure that we have the appropriate supports available to assist them.

## Duty of Care versus Legislation

Pharmacists have a duty of care to respond and assist their communities. This extends to times of great need, like emergencies and disasters. For many pharmacists, this places them in a difficult position to balance their duty of care obligations within the legal constraints of their jurisdiction. It becomes a tug-of-war between their ethical and moral responsibilities and the regulations and legislation that they are needing to work within. A study I conducted in 2018 reviewed pharmacy legislation that enabled pharmacists' roles in disasters for five countries.[3] It found with pharmacy legislation being state/provincial/jurisdiction based, there

DOI: 10.4324/b23292-20

was inconsistency in the pharmacy disaster-specific legislation that could be enacted during a state-declared emergency. However, the study did find a statistically significant association with the number of disasters that a jurisdiction experiences and the likelihood of them having disaster-specific pharmacy legislation.[3] They found that the more disaster events experienced by a jurisdiction the greater the odds of having disaster-specific emergency supply legislation and disaster-specific pharmacy relocation or mobile pharmacy legislation.[3]

### Disaster-Specific Emergency Supply Legislation

Under half of the jurisdictions studied had temporary legislation available to be enacted to increase the quantity of emergency medicine supplies from 3-days to 30-days.[3] But why is this so important? Below is a quote from an incident command controller that helps paint the picture of why this legislation is important.

> *We could have events where we get a couple of thousand tourists stranded. They come up just before the snow ... The roads are closed. They didn't bring any more medication than one night's worth or all the rest is left at home. But you go and see a chemist. We've actually had that one. So, I think in terms of providing pharmaceutical resupplies to transients like emergency services people, evacuees, tourists, there's a role there [for pharmacists]. [A1]*[4]

Some countries allow pharmacists to assist in short-term emergencies by using a 3-day emergency supply rule to ensure the continuity of medication supply.[5,6] This rule enables pharmacists to supply medications at their discretion to individuals who do not have a valid prescription and when the pharmacist is unable to contact the prescriber for authorisation in circumstances where not supplying a medication could lead to patient harm.[5] Under this rule, in everyday individual emergencies, pharmacists are able to provide a patient with a 3-day supply of their regular ongoing medication or a single dosing unit of devices for products such as insulin pens, inhalers, or creams.[5,6] A 3-day supply was initially introduced because this number of days covered a patient over weekends and public holidays and allowed them time to arrange a physician's appointment for a new prescription.[7,8] A clinical audit in England found patients most often accessing community pharmacies for an emergency supply were elderly patients requiring refills of their long-term chronic condition medications.[7] Allowing pharmacists to provide emergency supplies was found to reduce the burden on other areas of the healthcare system, including after-hours general practitioners and hospitals.[7]

To address population-wide disruptions, a state of emergency or disaster can be declared by a government. Due to the significant community service disruptions that occur during a disaster, the 3-day emergency supply rule is not generally adequate because it can take community services longer than three days to return to operational.[6] Some jurisdictions have recognised this and have adopted emergency supply legislation specific to statedeclared disasters.[3,8] This legislation gives pharmacists the authority to provide a longer emergency supply to patients, with some regions allowing up to 30-days supply.[3,8,9] This could alleviate some of the healthcare burden during disasters from lower-acuity patients crowding tertiary hospitals and emergency departments requiring refills of their chronic condition medications, freeing up doctors' and nurses' time to treat the disaster emergencies. In 2018, the pharmacy legislation review study found that the majority of the jurisdictions did not have this rule available to be enacted.[3]

For pharmacists not in prescribing regions or that do not have the 30-day emergency ruling, they are bound by this 3-day legislation and they discuss the compounding trauma for patients required to come back every three days and the increased workload and burden on them to continually provide small quantities of medicines. Therefore, more often in a disaster, pharmacists find themselves spending hours attempting to contact and get prescriptions from patients' doctors from other states to be able to provide an adequate supply of medications. Pharmacists sometimes find themselves considering providing patients with what is colloquially called an 'owing' for a month's supply of their medications to get them through the crisis until they can get to their doctor to obtain a prescription to cover the 'owing' provided. Some pharmacists consider supplying an 'owing' prescription for medications to continue the care of patients is ethically appropriate. However, this supply of a month's worth of medications without a prescription is not allowed according to many jurisdictions' pharmacy legislation.

Of course, there are some jurisdictions that have prescribing pharmacists that negate the need for this rule but not all pharmacists in all regions have their prescribing authority and their communities would still benefit from this temporary legislation. For example, while the province of Alberta in Canada has prescribing pharmacists, this is not true in other Canadian provinces and territories.[10]

### Disaster-Specific Relocation and Mobile Pharmacy Legislation

Let's look at another enabling piece of pharmacy legislation that the 2018 study reviewed. In a disaster, a pharmacy's premises may be damaged and not be safe for operations. However, this does not mean the pharmacist and pharmacy staff cannot assist their communities. There are two legislation options that can be enacted during a declared state of emergency or disaster for pharmacists to continue operating their pharmacy:

(1) take mobile pharmacies into a disaster zone operating under the licence of an existing premises; or (2) suspend their licence and temporarily relocate their premises to a new facility (usually for no longer than six months). It depends on the country as to which legislative option is preferred. In Australia, pharmacies are approved by both state and federal government legislation. They are able to apply for temporary relocation to continue providing services until their original premises are operational again under the Federal government National Health Act 1953.[11] In the United States, pharmacies typically operate mobile pharmacies from their existing premises into disaster zones.[12] Another recent study found that while the disaster health community may be accepting of pharmacists undertaking more clinical roles in disasters, a significant barrier of legislation was identified.[13]

A recent study exploring pharmacists' roles during the 2019-2020 Black Summer Bushfires in Australia found that pharmacists in evacuated towns were instructed to remain operational by local authorities.[14] Additionally, they identified the challenge with pharmacy legislation that mandated medications be dispensed from a licensed pharmacy.[14] This caused a barrier for the pharmacists working with the evacuation centres and forced them to work remotely from the local doctors within the centre and spend valuable time driving to and from the pharmacy to the evacuation centre.[14]

## Other Issues

An interesting point regarding legality of medication supply during disasters and emergencies was raised by a disaster pharmacist who has extensive experience in the field.

> *It kind of amazed me that in a regular hospital or a retail setting nothing happens that isn't supervised by a pharmacist. That's the law in most places here and yet they [disaster teams] were sending medicines out into the field completely unsupervised which would be enough to lose your pharmacy licence in the real world. [19]*[4]

Another ethical consideration that has been raised in the emergency management space is the giving away of free medications in a disaster. In many instances, patients cannot pay for them as they have been evacuated without their money or with power outages electronic payment methods are not operational and can be down for days to weeks. This places pharmacists in a difficult position as their duty of care of do no harm indicates the medication is needed and yet, regulations prohibit the free distribution of medications. Additionally, for regions that have insurance systems that cover the cost of medications, there are challenges with time taken to contact insurers and obtain approval to provide the medication. For example, there are limits on how frequently people can refill a prescription, so in an emergency if a patient leaves their home without taking their newly filled bottle of pills with them, they can struggle to get more supply (covered by insurance) as they are within the prohibited refill window. While pharmacists may be able to advocate on a patient's behalf given the extenuating circumstances of the disaster, this takes time. That's often time pharmacists responding in an emergency don't necessarily have and would be better served directly working with their patients and not on the phone.

## Government Involvement

There is a role for pharmacists to play assisting governments to improve their health emergency plans. Government and health departments tend to have a narrow view on healthcare services and the immediate professionals necessary to provide them. They often overlook the community services (i.e. family physician practices and pharmacies) and focus on the emergency services and government funded hospitals. Pharmacy professional organisations should be advocating, promoting, and raising awareness of pharmacists' roles in disasters and pharmacists should be given the opportunity to contribute on health policy decisions especially in terms of emergency management as they make up a significant portion of the private health sector assisting the community.

It has also been suggested that there is a need for governments to support pharmacists' roles in emergencies. Pharmacists working on the frontlines should be consulted throughout the PPRR cycle to ensure the health response outlined by the government is feasible and utilises pharmacists' skills and full scope of practice. For example, with the COVID-19 pandemic frontline pharmacists were not consulted regarding the COVID testing and vaccinations to be conducted in community pharmacies. Specifically, regarding the changing eligibility requirements for COVID vaccinations. Many pharmacists reported the lack of transparency and communication from the government and their professional organisations, claiming their patients were told about the changes via the media before the pharmacists that were actually providing the service.

## Chapter References

1 Haggan M. *Pharmacists battle to help patients [Internet]*. AJP News: Australian Journal of Pharmacy (AJP); 2019 [cited 2019 7th Feb]; Available from: http://www.webcitation.org/76KrFnTxt
2 Jackson A. *Pharmacist uses snowmobile to deliver medicine for snowed-in customers [Internet]*. CNN Health: CNN; 2019 [cited 2019 7th Feb]; Available from: http://www.webcitation.org/76Kr5Jgiz

3 Watson KE, Singleton JA, Tippett V, Nissen LM Do disasters predict international pharmacy legislation?. *Aust. Health Rev.* 2019; 44:392–398.

4 Watson KE *The Roles of Pharmacists in Disaster Health Management in Natural and Anthropogenic Disasters.* [Thesis]. QUT ePrints: Queensland University of Technology; 2019 Available from: https://eprints.qut.edu.au/130757/

5 Department of Health, Government of Western Australia. Emergency Supply of Medicines. Medicines and Poisons Regulation Branch; [cited 2019 -04-02]; Available from: https://ww2.health.wa.gov.au/Articles/A_E/Emergency-supply-of-medicines

6 Pharmaceutical Guild of Australia. Medicine Access in Emergencies [Internet]. Pharmaceutical Guild of Australia; 2019 [cited 2019-04-05]; Available from: https://www.guild.org.au/news-events/news/forefront/v09n03/medicine-access-in-emergencies

7 Morecroft CW, Mackridge AJ, Stokes EC, Gray NJ, Wilson SE, Ashcroft DM, et al. Emergency Supply of Prescription-Only Medicines to Patients by Community Pharmacists: A Mixed Methods Evaluation Incorporating Patient, Pharmacist and GP Perspectives. *BMJ Open* 2015; 5(7).

8 Kim J A Review of State Emergency Prescription Refill Protocols [Internet]. Healthcare Ready2014 [cited 2017-06-22]; Available from: http://www.webcitation.org/76KqNGucr

9 Ford H, Trent S, Wickizer S An Assessment of State Board of Pharmacy Legal Documents for Public Health Emergency Preparedness. *Am. J. Pharm. Educ.* 2016; 80(2).

10 Canadian Pharmacists Association. Pharmacists' Scope of Practice in Canada [Internet]. 2016 [cited 2018-08-07]; Available from: http://www.webcitation.org/76Kr06Aeg

11 Office of Parliamentary Counsel. National Health Act 1953. Canberra, Australia; 2018. p. 122–126.

12 California State Board of Pharmacy. 2019 Lawbook for Pharmacy. Business and Professions Code Chapter 9 Division 2 Section 4062. 2019. p. 53–54.

13 Watson KE, Tippett V, Singleton JA, Nissen LM Disaster Health Management: Do Pharmacists Fit in the Team? *Prehosp. Disaster Med.* 2019; 34(1):30–37.

14 Moss A, Green T, Moss S, Waghorn J, Bushell MJ Exploring Pharmacists' Roles during the 2019-2020 Australian Black Summer Bushfires. *Pharmacy (Basel)* 2021; 9(3).

# 17 How to Prepare for Disasters and Emergencies as Pharmacists and Pharmacy Students

## Introduction

Now that we have established the importance of our role as pharmacists in disasters and emergencies, I imagine many of you are wondering 'what to do' or 'where to start'. A quote I read from an article has stuck with me ever since and it says, *"The belief that pharmacists can simply rise to the occasion when it occurs is both naïve and dangerous and will likely leave us standing on the sidelines watching in frustration"*.[1] We have already covered what preparedness means as part of the PPRR cycle and the importance of it. So, together in this chapter we will walk through some of the beginnings of how to approach preparedness and where to begin. In the following chapter, we will cover how to train and teach our colleagues, teams, students, and staff for disasters and emergencies.

Preparedness is crucial because without proper preparedness our response will be inappropriate. It is not up to others to dictate the pharmacy workforce's emergency response. However, others will step in and tell us how pharmacy should respond in the absence of us and our profession having detailed plans and routinely undertaking preparedness activities. This has been seen in countless previous disasters and was evident during the COVID-19 pandemic.

Please note this doesn't mean that only pharmacists in management style positions or those that deploy to regions impacted by disasters should be prepared, but I am referring to every individual pharmacist. Every pharmacist ... is a disaster and public health pharmacist, regardless of your practice setting.

## Personal Preparedness

So, how do we get personally prepared for a disaster or emergency. First, it is a good idea to know the specific risks of your environment where you live and work. For example, do you live near a fault line that increases the risk of earthquakes? Are hurricanes or cyclones common in your region? Is your work or home on a floodplain? By asking these types of questions

DOI: 10.4324/b23292-21

we can begin to appreciate the risks and put our plans in place. We should still be considering taking an all-hazard approach to our plans as we have discussed earlier in this book, but it is helpful to know the specific risks in the region as well. For example, in the story I shared about my personal experience of a disaster in Chapter 1. I should have known about the increased likelihood of flash floods following storms in my area.

Secondly, you need to have your own plan as we cannot rely on others to develop one for us or our response could be inappropriate to the needs around us. The key step in emergency management is not in the response but in being better prepared. So, let me ask you some questions to get you started but I encourage you to explore your local resources (e.g., government websites, NGOs, local organisations, etc.) to help you build your own plan and your family's plan.

- Are you willing to respond to an emergency impacting your community?
- Do you have an emergency go bag packed?
- Do you have an emergency kit and supplies to be self-sufficient if you are required to shelter at home for several days?
- Do you have a list of important contacts?
- Do you have a reserve of chronic condition medications?
- Have you and your family practiced evacuation routes?
- Do you have a planned location to meet up, if you are not together as a family when evacuated and the telecommunications are down?
- If a disaster impacts your community, will you turn up to work when you are not rostered?
- In the event you need to work during an emergency, have you considered childcare or caring arrangements for the people you support?
- Will you restrict your working hours? Will you increase them to meet a need?
- Would you change your response depending on the type of emergency event?

This is not an exhaustive list, but it is a good place to start thinking about how you want to be personally prepared for a disaster. If you don't know your answer to some of these, I encourage you to start now on the backside of the COVID-19 pandemic, what lessons have your learnt that can be incorporated into a personal preparedness plan for the next emergency? As it is not a matter of 'if' we have another one but when, how, and what actions we are prepared to take.

## Selfcare

When it comes to disasters and emergencies, it would be naïve of us to overlook the simple fact that we are human beings as well as healthcare professionals. While that may seem like a straightforward statement, just stop for a minute and read the statement again – we are human beings as well as healthcare professionals. We as pharmacists are notorious for putting everyone else – our patients, staff, clients, and colleagues before ourselves. So much so that a prideful statement often uttered by pharmacists is "*I can hold it, I'm a pharmacist*", implying that pharmacists have a superpower of forgoing the need to go to the bathroom as the phone is ringing and people are waiting on us that we can't possibly take the two minutes to go to the toilet.

While I applaud the selflessness of our profession, I am also concerned by it when it comes to disasters and emergencies as it can and has in the past become our Achilles heel. I am not saying this is a bad quality as it shows the heart that pharmacists have for their patients and community. But it can become self-limiting during emergencies, as they are high stress environments and if we do not take care of ourselves, we cannot take care of others. So, I am here to remind you and myself that we make better clinical decisions and are better at focusing on our patients when we aren't tired, hungry, or needing to use the bathroom. So, let's talk about selfcare for a minute.

Selfcare is not selfish. Let me repeat that for us … **selfcare is not selfish!**

Do you recall the safety briefing given by flight attendants before the plane takes off … ? Something to the effect of "*In the event of an emergency, oxygen masks will appear above you. It is important you place your own mask on before helping others*". I believe the same applies to us as healthcare professionals and just basic humans. I am here to reinforce this message for you for when you are responding and recovering from an emergency. If you do not practice selfcare then you are putting yourself and your patients' safety at risk.

So, what is selfcare … essentially think of what we tell our patients but are not so good at doing ourselves? Small but effective measures we can take could include:

- Take bathroom breaks
- Take lunch and food breaks
- Debrief with your team
- Find ways to de-stress on the way home from work (e.g., listening to a funny podcast, relaxing music, or chatting to a friend)
- Prioritise your tasks and give yourself permission not to get to everything
- Understand and accept that unfortunately, we can't do everything on the to-do list. All we can do is to try our best each day, and that's enough!
- Try to set firm boundaries. Don't bring work home with you, don't work on your days off, and take your 'helper hat' off when you're talking to friends and family

- Take time each day to work out what you need. It could be more social interaction, to move your body more, or time for stillness and rest
- Engage with hobbies
- Get adequate sleep and rest
- Notice how you're eating, how much water you're drinking, and whether your mind is racing

This is not an exhaustive list but a few things I believe are applicable to us as pharmacists. It's a good place to start and if you notice changes in your sleep, eating habits, or the way you interact with people you care about, it would be a good idea to stop and check in to see how you're feeling and coping. I would encourage you to take time to write your own selfcare plan of things that are specific to you and take advantages of the resources that are available.

Debriefing is encouraged and effective to help us process with people that experienced the same circumstances or situation. This is not rehashing the event or playing the blame game but talking through with those that were present about the challenges you experienced and brainstorming solutions moving forward for next time. A word of caution, be mindful of who you choose to debrief with. Debriefing to loved ones can be challenging as they were not present and can sometimes experience vicarious trauma through your stories.

## Professional Preparedness

Being prepared as healthcare professionals is essential because if we have a prepared health workforce this would result in a resilient workforce that is willing, capable, and safe to practice effectively in an emergency response to a disaster.[2] Currently, there is little focus on preparedness of pharmacists and pharmacy staff, with any existing literature being specific to preparing pharmacies.[3] However, this line of thinking overlooks the key concept that – to have a prepared pharmacy capable of responding during a disaster, there needs to be prepared pharmacists and pharmacy staff to make it operational.[3] A study conducted in Australia found that pharmacists that feel a professional responsibility to respond in a disaster are more likely to engage in preparedness behaviours and be more willing to work during an emergency.[2,3] So, let's look at some ways in which we can become professionally prepared.

## Continuing Professional Development

Disaster and emergency preparedness is not a 'one and done' kind of training but it is something we should be continually working on and training in. Presently, there is limited tailored education and training available for pharmacists to undertake specific to disaster and emergency management. This is something that I am hoping will change in the post-COVID era and is the reason I started my business – Disaster Pharmacy Solutions™. Our vision is to build a pharmacy workforce that is: (1) equipped to handle unexpected disasters or emergencies (e.g., COVID-19 pandemic, floods, fires, etc.); (2) confident to lead their communities through disasters and emergencies; and (3) trained in disaster planning and emergency management. I would encourage you to reach out to your professional organisations and universities in your region and begin advocating for education and continuing professional development in disaster management and emergency response. There are some opportunities beginning to appear, like the online American Society of Health-System Pharmacists 'Crisis and Pandemic Management Certificate', which I contributed to and became available in 2021 in response to the needs of pharmacists responding to the COVID-19 pandemic.[4]

Pharmacists would benefit from generic disaster and emergency management courses and trainings as well as tailored pharmacy courses. For example, psychological first aid training, hazardous materials training, major incident medical management and support training, national incident management training, etc. Many governments and organisations offer these trainings and some are available online and free of charge (e.g., Federal Emergency Management Agency (FEMA) Independent Study Program,[5] WHO online courses[6]).

In the next chapter, we will discuss teaching and preparedness training in more detail.

## After-Action Reports and Reviews

We've covered in this book the PPRR cycle and discussed how the phases are overlapping and continuous, so in reality we do not start with prevention or preparedness but actually start from the recovery of the previous event. We need to learn from lessons and challenges of the current event as we prepare for the next. To do this, we engage in debriefing and after-action reviews/reports. These reviews or reports don't need to be anything fancy, but a simple process undertaken by you and your team to answer the following types of questions,

1   What was expected to occur?
2   What actually happened?
3   What went wrong and why?
4   What went well and why?
5   What needs to be changed for next time?

By going through this process, it allows everyone to review the thought-processes and decision-making using the glorious hindsight. It is designed to be a learning tool and not an activity in blaming people for errors or mistakes but ensuring that they are not repeated in future incidences. We can learn from the past and use it to inform our future directions.

## Chapter References

1 Klepser ME. Seasonal and pandemic influenza: Preparing pharmacists for the frontline. *J. Am. Pharm. Assoc.* (2003) 2008; 48(2):312–314.

2 McCourt EM. *Australian pharmacists' preparedness to fulfil roles in disasters and emergencies [Thesis].* QUT ePrints: Queensland University of Technology; 2019.

3 McCourt EM, Singleton JA, Tippett V, Nissen LM. Evaluation of disaster preparedness and preparedness behaviors among pharmacists: A cross-sectional study in Australia. *Prehosp. Disaster Med.* 2021; 36(3):354–361.

4 American Society of Health-System Pharmacists. *Crisis and pandemic management certificate.* eLearning: ASHP; 2021 [cited 2022 June 27]; Available from: https://elearning.ashp.org/products/8799/crisis-and-pandemic-management-certificate

5 FEMA Emergency Management Institute. *FEMA independent study (IS) program: Distance learning: ISP courses [Internet].* FEMA; 2020 [cited 2022 June 27]; Available from: https://training.fema.gov/is/crslist.aspx

6 World Health Organization. *OpenWHO – Courses [Internet].* WHO; [cited 2022 June 27]; Available from: https://openwho.org/courses

# 18 Teaching Disaster and Emergency Management in Pharmacy School

## Introduction

Disaster preparedness activities are important in their own right but they also have the added benefits of being a medium in which to teach and practice other skills (e.g. leadership, autonomy, teamwork, problem-solving, communication, etc.). All of these skills are vital to being a healthcare professional and working to your fullest as a pharmacist or pharmacy team member.

Disasters are unique circumstances that stripe away ourthe ability to rely on technology and removes some of the luxuries we depend on in our everyday practices. It eliminates the crutch we sometimes have on being able to offload decision-making to other healthcare professionals and our natural default of risk-aversion or avoidance pressing us to step into our full scope of practice in the best interests of our patients. For example, in a power outage; we must think through the need to manage controlled substances, the legal requirements for handwritten labels, or manually checking drug interactions. Tasks that are normally so easily managed using our electronic systems within our departments and pharmacies.

I believe in building a resilient pharmacy workforce that can be relied upon to be active participants in local disaster and health response teams. People I have worked with and those that have participated in our research studies state they would like more opportunities to learn and practice their disaster PPRR plans and roles. So, I believe there is a hunger and appetite among the pharmacy workforce for disaster focused professional development opportunities, especially on the tailend of the COVID-19 pandemic.

Research has highlighted the need for universities to incorporate education on disaster and emergency management including decision-making models.[1] During disasters with the absence of other healthcare professionals to delegate to or rely on, the needs of patients pushes the scale and encourages pharmacists to move up the hierarchical model for decision-making. It is suggested there are four levels to decision-making models: submissive, corrective, consultive, and prescriptive. Emergencies

DOI: 10.4324/b23292-22

sees us as pharmacists shift from submissive to prescriptive in our decision-making and from passive to active management.[1] This can be observed in the earlier chapters where we reviewed previous disaster and emergency events and how pharmacists step up to meet the needs of their communities. So, it's important that our education and trainings support and encourage this change in decision-making. On another note, it is important that we as pharmacists understand the 'do no harm' principles in context of emergency events. Recall the story shared in Chapter 15 by Capt. Tim Davis about ensuring healthcare professionals work not only within their scope but also within the bounds of their environmental context.

These skills should be taught within our pharmacy education and routinely provided in continuing professional development opportunities, to ensure that our workforce is resilient and prepared to undertake their vital role in a disaster or emergency. The earlier sections of this book can be used to teach the fundamentals and basics about disaster and emergency management and this chapter complements this with an application-based exercise and guidance to run interactive workshops. In addition to this, it is felt that disaster activities are important for all prospective pharmacists and pharmacy staff to participate and train in. Remember, we can utilise our pharmacy staff and students to backfill roles and free up pharmacists' time for other emergency roles.

In 2019, my team and I conducted a research study evaluating the confidence and preparedness of Australian pharmacists pre- and post- a disaster preparedness workshop held during a national conference.[2] What we found was that 87.8% of those that attended and completed the surveys believed the workshop improved their understanding of disaster management activities; 90.2% believed the exercise helped them to identify their strengths as well as any gaps in their understanding of disaster preparedness, response, and recovery; and 92.7% wanted more learning opportunities specific to emergency management.[2]

## Mass Gathering Medicine

One way for pharmacists to train and prepare for disasters and emergencies, is to participate in mass gathering medicine. We discussed this in Chapter 14 as an enabler for pharmacists' roles in disasters and emergencies. This can be either through formal participation or in the absence of being able to formally take part in these activities, individual pharmacists, departments, or pharmacies can take time to internally workshop their emergency plan for a mass gathering event. For example, would your department or pharmacy extend their operating hours in the event of an emergency taking place at the event? What steps would you need to take if the security of your premise is compromised? Below is a story that was shared with me by a United States pharmacist about how valuable pharmacists and pharmacy students can be in mass gathering medicine.

*Okay, so it's a 3:30pm game at the Stadium. There are 95,000 people there. It's hot and it's September. It's probably 98 degrees outside and about 98% humidity. There are literally hundreds of people coming to the first aid stations that we have. We have four cooling buses set up outside the stadium that people can go out and just sit in so they can cool off and they're full. The first aid stations are overrun with people with heat exhaustion and alcohol because people drink before they come to the game. They don't realise how much they've drank and then they get dehydrated on top of it. We have a young woman in one of the first aid stations. She comes in. She's obviously drunk. She's probably a little dehydrated. They get her in, they give her some fluids, they get an IV [intravenous] and they say that she probably needs to stay a little longer, but they really don't have a lot of space for her. So, she decides that she's going to leave, and she'll be fine. She gets up to leave and starts to walk out of the first aid station.*

*One of my pharmacy students notices that on her thong, because her clothes are a little dishevelled, there's a black box that looks like a pager. And the pharmacy student says "wait a second! before you go, I want you to come sit back down" and then they inform the paramedic she has an insulin pump. So, the paramedic says, "oh my god" and they do a blood glucose and her blood glucose is 536 mg/dL [~30 mmol/L]. She starts to lose some of her faculties... So, they put her in the ambulance and take her down there but none of that would have happened had my student not noticed the fact that the woman was wearing an insulin pump.*

*I don't think just anybody would have recognised it for what it was and that's the difference of someone who just has a little bit of a knowledge, and a little bit of observation skill can make with someone. The paramedics were going to let her walk out because they didn't know, but my student did. [15]*[3]

## An Evolving Emergency Scenario – Worked Example

Before beginning to design a scenario, it's important to reflect your purpose. Some questions to consider are:

- What are the learning outcomes you are wanting to achieve?
- What is the knowledge level of your students or participants?
- How much time do you have? (don't forget you need to incorporate time for debriefing and discussion)
- Are there additional skills you want to include (e.g. leadership, teamwork, communication, etc.)?

I have included in this book, a worked example that was designed for third year pharmacy students to open up conversations about and to introduce to disaster management and emergency response. It has been modified slightly for this book's readership. This scenario is hypothetical and has been created to be as real as possible, but the places, names, and events are fictional and only for educational purposes.

These types of activities are best undertaken in small teams and the below worked example would take approximately three hours to complete including a time for debrief and discussion. While it can be tempting to skip the debrief and discussion if you are short on time, I would strongly caution against this. As it is in the debrief and discussion that the learning is consolidated, and you are individually enriched from the group discussion. I've been running these sessions for several years in different educational programs and conferences and I have always come away with new understanding and perspective from the people and participants I work with. It depends on the size of your group that you are working with and their level of comprehension regarding these types of disaster preparedness activities, to how long it would take and how much time should be dedicated to the debrief and discussion.

### *The Scenario Begins ...*

You are attending a pharmacy conference being held in a small fictional city of Wellington (population 2.5 million). There hasn't been much rain during the summer and the fire danger is high, but no one is overly concerned at this time.

**Day 1:** You wake up early to attend the conference breakfast. While sharing breakfast in the hotel with your colleagues the conference organisers make an announcement,

> *Due to the wind activity a small fire has started in the nearby National Park. Currently there is no risk to us here and we will continue with the conference as scheduled.*

**Day 2:** The wind has changed direction and the forest fire has moved rapidly through the dry vegetation and into the National Park. A voluntary evacuation call has been made and everyone at the conference are relocating to the nearby larger city of Ryantowne. The local health services in Ryantowne are severely understaffed and their emergency plans were recently destroyed as they were located in a basement which recently experienced a flooding event. The local government heard the conference was in town and have requested assistance from the conference coordinators and delegates.

It is estimated that 500 people from the city of Wellington will be relocating to the evacuation centre being set up in Ryantowne. Some people may need to stay there for as long as a week. The evacuation centre is being set up in the recreation centre which has the following facilities – bathrooms (10 cubicles), showers (4), running water, electricity is currently working, sheds in back, open grassy area, lockable storage rooms (usually sporting equipment kept there).

Complete Activity 1.

*Activity 1: In your teams, make a list of what items might be needed in the evacuation centre and consider the following three categories*

1   *Facility Needs (e.g., power)*
2   *Operational Needs (e.g., phone access)*
3   *Welfare Needs (e.g., water)*

**Day 3:** The organisers know that a lot of different people are going to be coming to the evacuation centre (young families, the elderly, minors, people by themselves, people requiring additional assitance, etc.) and they are all going to have different medical needs. Some will require no medical treatment, some might have obtained acute injuries in the fire, and others might need their regular medications.

Because the emergency plans were destroyed, the evacuation centre coordinators have asked your team to create a 'triage tool' to determine an efficent way of assessing the needs of the disaster-affected individuals and identifying how different healthcare professionals can help best meet their needs.

Complete Activity 2.

*Activity 2: In your group, design a triage tool that could be used to assess the needs of disaster-affected individuals and that utilises the healthcare professionals you have available, most effectively. Also consider if there are any additional health professionals you would like to collaborate with in the emergency response?*
    *Volunteering at the evacuation centre are:*

- *6 pharmacists*
- *2 nurses*
- *1 family physician*
- *1 nurse practitioner*
- *2 paramedic / EMT*
- *1 dietician*
- *1 social worker*
- *a few of the disaster-affected individuals attending the evacuation centre have offered to help out where needed*

**Day 3 cont'd:** Now that your team has developed your triage tool, the coordinators have asked you to 'test run' your triage/patient flow tool on some people that are waiting to come into the centre, before the bus loads of evacuees will arrive that afternoon.

As a team, reflect on the effectiveness of your tool, identify any gaps in the system, and adapt your tool as required.

Complete Activity 3.

*Activity 3:* Now that in your teams you have developed your triage/patient flow tool, it is time to test its effectiveness on some incoming evacuees. For each individual evacuee, note and discuss how your tool would assess them as they are coming into the recreation centre. What services or professionals might they require?

> Sally Rogers is a 45-year-old woman who has chronic obstructive pulmonary disease. Sally has presented to the evacuation centre from work and does not know where her partner (they were at work) or children (they are in daycare) are as the power lines are down. She currently uses two inhalers once a day and uses a CPAP machine to sleep at night.

> Timothy Cambridge has arrived at the evacuation centre; he seems agitated, pale, and struggling to catch his breath after rushing here from helping to evacuate his neighbours from his building to the evacuation centre. When asking him to complete the entry survey, you notice that he has burns to his forearms and upper arms. Timothy was not aware of the burns and does not seem to feel them.

> The Browns are a family of three - single mother with a 3-year-old and a 6-month-old (being bottled-fed). They have presented at the evacuation centre after fleeing from their home. They only have the clothes on their backs and the 3-year-old's teddy bear which is a little singed from the fire. The 3-year-old has acute otitis media (you can see them tugging at their ear, they have a slight fever, and are noticeably irritable) and has been given amoxicillin to treat.

> Bonus Question: The 3-year-old (14 kgs, 30.87 lbs) that has acute otitis media and was given amoxicillin 8.4mLs of a 250 mg/5 mL preparation three times a day for 5 days. Are there any issues with this?

**Day 4:** The items that you have requested have been set up in the centre. Disaster-affected individuals are arriving, and your patient flow and triage tool is being used to assess their health needs.

The coordinators come to you concerned, as they are worried about so many people in a close space using the same facilities that this could contribute to an infectious disease outbreak. They have requested you launch a public health campaign to help educate the evacuees in the centre on some important health measures.

Complete Activity 4.

*Activity 4:* *There is a concern of an infection outbreak at the evacuation centre with so many people in a confined space. In your teams, develop a brief public health campaign poster to encourage the evacuees to practice better hygiene (e.g. handwashing, etc.).*

**Debrief:** Now move into a debrief and discussion time. I recommend having time for each small group to debrief together and then bringing it together as a large group.

## Chapter References

1 Moss A, Green T, Moss S, Waghorn J, Bushell MJ. Exploring pharmacists' roles during the 2019-2020 Australian black summer bushfires. *Pharmacy (Basel)* 2021; 9(3).
2 Watson KE, Waddell JJ, McCourt EM. "Vital in today's": Evaluation of a disaster table-top exercise for pharmacists and pharmacy staff. *Research in Social and Administrative Pharmacy* 2021; 17(5):858–863. doi: 10.1016/j.sapharm.2020.07.009.
3 Watson KE. *The roles of pharmacists in disaster health management in natural and anthropogenic disasters.* [Thesis]. QUT ePrints: Queensland University of Technology; 2019 Available from: https://eprints.qut.edu.au/130757/.

# 19 Disasters and Emergencies that Change Us

## Introduction

We have reviewed the history and evolution of pharmacists' roles in disasters and emergencies in Chapter 6. While every previous event has led to a small positive change for our profession in disaster management, none have made as big as an impact as the most recent COVID-19 pandemic. In this chapter, we explore this impact in detail and its ripple effects that have occurred across the profession. This global disaster has not only impacted in the obvious ways, like how we have adapted our pharmacy roles and services. But it has also changed how we see ourselves as pharmacists and how we view the profession. Research suggests we are on the precipice of a new era for pharmacy practice.

Disasters and emergencies are stressful and chaotic events that can fundamentally change who we are. Pharmacists' experiences of the changes in their roles while responding to the needs of society during the COVID-19 pandemic may have implications for their professional role identity.[1] We theorise that the COVID-19 pandemic with the global impact of this crisis and the prolonged need for these adaptive and innovative pharmacists' roles and services – that this is acting as a catalyst for pharmacists' professional role identity change.[1] We also suggest that there is an 'invisible layer' of change occurring in the pharmacy profession as a ripple effect of the pandemic.[1] The ongoing nature and global scale of this pandemic has required continued adaption of pharmacists' roles and services and perhaps this has led to long-lasting professional role changes and our understanding of our evolving professional identities.[1]

## Professional Role Identity

Professional roles, expressed as professional identity, shape who pharmacists are, what they do, and what they stand for as professionals.[1] The relationship between professional roles and identity are intimately related. Roles represent a social prescription for behaviour, whereas identity is an

DOI: 10.4324/b23292-23

internal self-understanding of the professional role.[2] Professional role identity represents how professionals see themselves in relation to their professional roles: who they are and how they should act.[3,4] Professional role identity is dynamic. Changes in work role are among the many contributors to changes in professional role identity.[1] The COVID-19 pandemic presents an opportunity for pharmacists to see themselves through the essential roles that they have performed, acting as a mirror in which pharmacists can see their reflection of their various roles and evolving professional role identity.[1] Through the lens of professional role identity,[3,4] perhaps the prolonged nature and demands of COVID-19 has been the catalyst to the new equilibrium of pharmacy practice change and pharmacists' professional role identity.

## New Era of Pharmacy Practice

Nadeem and colleagues have suggested there has been a paradigm shift of pharmacists' roles to a focus on patient care, as a trusted information source with greater autonomy because of the COVID-19 pandemic.[5] This sentiment is echoed by Hayden and colleagues, who believe the pandemic will push the pharmacy profession into a 'new era' of pharmacy practice.[6] Additionally, the recent scoping review conducted by our team also supports this idea and expanded it with our conceptual framework model proposing that the pandemic is leading to a new equilibrium for sustainable pharmacists' professional role changes and which we call the 'invisible layer' of change.[1]

## The PRINT Working Theory: Professional Role Identity in Transition

The concept of an 'invisible layer' of change led to my team's new study (IGNITE) that is currently underway and is funded by the Canadian Foundation for Pharmacy.[7] We aim to evaluate the influence of the COVID-19 pandemic on pharmacists' professional roles and identity. We anticipate this study will answer two main questions; (1) How has the COVID-19 pandemic influenced pharmacists' roles and their professional identity (what they do and what it means to them)? and (2) Which aspects of pharmacists' roles and professional identity have changed, if any, and are they projected to be sustained post-COVID-19?[7]

This study is still underway, but our current working theory is that disasters and emergencies act as an external ignition point which forces a conscious exploration of our role and identity as pharmacists; essentially making the invisible layer of change that is occurring visible (Figure 19.1). For example, changes in public health policy made pharmacists' role in public health more visible and at the forefront of our minds. This forced the transition and the internal conscious

**The PRINT Theory: Professional Role Identity in Transition**

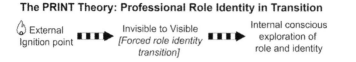

*Figure 19.1* The PRINT theory: Professional role identity in transition (a work in progress).

exploration of role identity (e.g., who am I as a pharmacist? and does this role/service I am performing fit with how I view myself as a pharmacist?). While these findings are specific to the COVID-19 pandemic, the implications of this theory can be further explored, as any external ignition point (e.g., change in practice setting or job or priorities) could result in the same internal conscious exploration of who we are and what we do. This internal exploration is how we settle the cognitive dissonance that we may experience when the role or service we are performing does not match with our role identity.

### Crisis Communication

We worked with a pharmacy resident to conduct a content analysis study reviewing the communications of pharmacy organisations during the first year of the COVID-19 pandemic for Alberta pharmacists.[8] What was surprising to discover with this study was that pharmacy organisations' crisis communication and direction that was provided to help pharmacists navigate the changing context of the COVID-19 pandemic emphasised pharmacists as information professionals and their roles in public health positioning them as a reliable source for COVID conversations. While pharmacists are information and drug experts, when we are faced with an unknown context (like the global pandemic), we revert to a novice proficiency level requiring additional instruction and guidance to help navigate our actions and respond to the new context. So, we need to support our frontline pharmacists in their roles during emergencies, by ensuring our communication is direct and clear. Miscommunications can occur if the pharmacy organisations' communications require inference as to what pharmacists are supposed to do. Crisis communication needs to be direct and timely as disasters do not give us the luxury of time to become comfortable before needing to respond.

### So, What's Next?

What we are beginning to discover is how influential this pandemic has been. While it has been a disaster in every sense of the word, I choose to find the silver lining in this tragedy. For me, it is the pride I see in my fellow pharmacists at the recognition that they were given being identified as essential and highly valued members in the emergency response.

The ripple effects of this pandemic and the full extent of its positive influences on our profession are still mostly unknown, but I am excited to embark on this new era of pharmacy practice with you and continue researching and writing our story together.

## Chapter References

1 Watson KE, Schindel TJ, Barsoum ME, Kung JY. COVID the catalyst for evolving professional role identity? A scoping review of global pharmacists' roles and services as a response to the COVID-19 pandemic. *Pharmacy* 2021; 9(2):99.

2 Simpson B, Carroll B. Re-viewing role in processes of identity construction. *Organization* 2008; 15(1):29–50.

3 Chreim S, Williams BE, Hinings CR. Interlevel influences on the reconstruction of professional role identity. *Acad. Manage. J.* 2007; 50(6):1515–1539.

4 Pratt MG, Rockmann KW, Kaufmann JB. Constructing professional identity: The role of work and identity learning cycles in the customization of identity among medical residents. *Acad. Manage. J.* 2006; 49(2):235–262.

5 Nadeem MF, Samanta S, Mustafa F. Is the paradigm of community pharmacy practice expected to shift due to COVID-19? *Res. Soc. Admin. Phar.* 2021; 17(1):2046–2048.

6 Hayden JC, Parkin R. The challenges of COVID-19 for community pharmacists and opportunities for the future. *Ir. J. Psychol. Med.* 2020; 37(3):198–203.

7 EPICORE Centre. COVID-19: Bringing the 'invisible layer' of pharmacists professional identity and roles to light (IGNITE) [Internet]. 2021 [cited 2022 July 7]; Available from: https://www.epicore.ualberta.ca/home/ignite/

8 Safnuk, C, Ackman, ML, Schindel, TJ, Watson, KE. The COVID Conversations: A content analysis of Canadian pharmacy organizations' communication of pharmacists' roles and services during the COVID-19 pandemic. *Can Pharm J.* 2022 (accepted for publication).

# 20 Conclusion

All pharmacists are disaster pharmacists!

This has become apparent to me over the years of researching in this field of disaster pharmacy. A lot of what we do during an emergency is an adaption of our everyday practice, however, it requires ongoing preparedness to ensure we feel confident and capable to step into the expectations placed on us. We need to be prepared and skilled in disaster management and emergency response to undertake our pivotal role in leading our communities through emergencies.

The pharmacy profession needs to be better integrated in disaster health management and have a seat at the table where disaster health decisions are made. I implore everyone reading this book to make some noise about how vital our pharmacists are during emergency response and disaster management. Together we can build on our experiences and learning from past disasters to help us prepare for the next crisis. As pharmacists we do not have to wait until we are in the thick of an emergency to risk actively engaging in the exploration of *what we do* or *how we act* in a disaster. Now is the time to start writing our lessons learnt, the after-action reports and reviews, and documenting the roles performed by our frontline pharmacists and the challenges they faced. We need to carry the momentum we have forward.

If we let this moment in history pass us by, we may lose out on the opportunity to reflect on how disasters change us as healthcare professionals and miss the opportunity to proactively chart permanent change for the profession.

This story is not over, and we have the power to write our own ending …

DOI: 10.4324/b23292-24

# Index

Note: **Bold** page numbers refer to tables and *italic* page numbers refer to figures.

Printed in the United States
by Baker & Taylor Publisher Services